Ex Libris

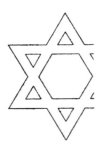

Anatoliy Usha
1927 – 2020
Leningrad, USSR –
Chicago,
IL, USA

Анатолий Уша
1927 – 2020 гг.
Ленинград, СССР –
Чикаго, Иллинойс,
США

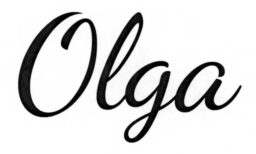

Olga

The *O.K.* Way to a
Healthy, Happy Life

By Olga Kotelko

With Roxanne Davies

Edited by Michele Carter

www.olgakotelko.com

Jacket design: Romy Ilich

Produced by:

FriesenPress

Suite 300 – 852 Fort Street

Victoria, BC, Canada V8W 1H8

www.friesenpress.com

Distributed to the trade by The Ingram Book Company

Contents

To the memory of my daughter, Nadine.

A Message to Readers

When Olga Kotelko asked if I would help to write a little book outlining her exercise program, which she called *The O.K. Way to a Healthy, Happy Life* immediately I said yes! Like so many other people, I wanted to know how this 95-year-old grandmother, who has been called one of the world's greatest athletes, achieves such remarkable physical accomplishments. After discussing the scope of the project, I suggested that Olga write a full account of her life. Happily she agreed.

As a newspaper reporter I was privileged to interview people of all ages. If the average lifespan is estimated to be 1000 months, Olga already has surpassed that number by 128 months, and she shows no signs of slowing down any time soon. While few of us can match Olga's extraordinary athletic prowess, I feel most of us can all learn some useful lessons from reading her story. Her message is simple. First and foremost: It's never too late to get on the road to physical fitness. Second: Have fun and don't act your age. Third: Make good choices and persevere. No cheating!

Olga's book is a richly woven fabric of colourful stories. She recounts her family life, her early career as a school teacher, and her many joys and challenges. Her straightforward and effective exercise and nutrition tips, which she explains in detail, will inform and motivate those readers who want to follow in her footsteps and embark on their own journey to health and well-being.

I've decided that when I grow up I want to be like Olga; I think we all do. She breathes self-confidence, and she has a passion and a zest for life that is utterly contagious. While we may not have been blessed with Olga's genes, we may want to emulate her physical, mental, and spiritual strategies for living a long, happy, and healthy life to the best of our abilities. Also, her story illustrates that you don't have to be a competitive athlete to create a healthy, happy lifestyle.

Olga writes, "These days, turning 60, 70, 80 and even 90 years of age will be nothing, if you take care of yourself, for nothing is beyond a woman or man's reach. . . . Old age isn't a disease any more than infancy. When it comes to health and wellness, seniors are not just part of the problem—we're actually part of the solution."

Olga's book is timely and inspiring. It contains her story as well as her opinions and ideas, and is intended to provide helpful information about her personal health regimen and what has worked for her. It is offered with the understanding that the author and publisher are not engaged in providing medical nor health services in the book. The reader should consult his or her doctor or other health professional before adopting any of the author's suggestions.

The author and publisher disclaim any responsibility for liability, loss, or risk that is incurred as a consequence, directly or indirectly, through the use or application of any of the contents of this book.

Roxanne Davies
Vancouver, BC
December 2013

Foreword

It was 2008, and I remember wondering if I was pushing my Aquafit participants just a little bit too hard. It was an Aquafit *Plus* class and the participants were mostly in their 60's and 70's. Was the cardio too fast? Was the strength just a bit too tough? I was reassured by several participants that it wasn't too hard, and I specifically remember a short, vibrant woman who approached me after class one day to let me know that this was good conditioning for a track and field meet she was participating in later that year. Imagine my surprise and disbelief when, about a year later, I found out Olga Kotelko was 90 years old and not the 70 or 80 that I had thought.

Several months after that initial conversation, she approached me to show me a number of gold medals she had won in a meet. It amazed me that this slight, spry 'old lady' could be that active and compete in events that most people would consider impossible for someone of her age. It was, and still is, inspiring to see this woman living such an active, vigorous life.

In the short time I have known Olga, I have watched as the world sat up and took notice of the 90-year old woman who wouldn't act her age. This active senior has been featured in magazines and on television, simply and quietly sharing her philosophies on activity and aging, and even sharing some of her training secrets. It has been a privilege to be even peripherally involved as Olga inspires and motivates those around her. She inspires and motivates me every day and has changed my ideas of what aging means. I know her words and story will inspire you too.

Daniel Godfrey
Aquatic Fitness Instructor
Aquatic Program Coordinator

As a medical practitioner, I have been in family medical practice since 1973. I have done extensive work in the Richmond Emergency Room and now have a special interest in geriatrics.

Olga Kotelko is a retired schoolteacher who has not taken the easy road to retirement. She challenged track and field after the age of 77 years, and she has been a force in the Masters category, competing locally, provincially, nationally, and internationally. She has achieved numerous records and won over 650 medals, the majority being gold, and she has led the Canadian contingent in international competition.

I have been aware of this amazing senior citizen's accomplishments for the last ten years and have been in awe of them. However, I am most impressed with her unassuming nature and matter-of-fact approach to the challenge of world competition.

She manages to train for these physically taxing events and still take an active part in her community, her Ukrainian Catholic Church and her family.

I organize and moderate continuing medical education courses for physicians and nurses in Vancouver and Richmond. Mrs. Kotelko has given freely of her time to come and address these events and act as an example to other seniors in the community to encourage them to maintain their own physical and mental fitness.

Michael Myckatyn, BA, MD

———————————

How is this little old lady going to keep up with us?

Shortly after I became the 3rd Ukrainian Catholic Bishop of New Westminster in the summer of 2007, I decided that I should try to visit all of the parishes in the Eparchy (Diocese). The Eparchy takes in all of British Columbia and Yukon, and although it is large in territory, there are fewer than 15 parishes. Olga Kotelko was one of the very first parishioners to sign up for the "August 2008 Pilgrimage to the Yukon with Bishop Ken".

When I first met her, she let me know that she, like me, was from Saskatchewan, and that she was almost 90 years old. I have to confess I was a bit nervous when I thought of having her on the pilgrimage. What if she couldn't keep up with the group? Who would stay behind with her? I placed my trust in God and in Olga.

My whole image of this short, elderly lady changed dramatically the first morning. Our little pilgrimage group arranged to meet in the hotel lobby for an early morning breakfast before heading out for a day of prayer and sight-seeing. I made sure that I was one of the first ones in the lobby; as group leader, I was expected to set a good example. I was not the first one down. In fact, it was Olga, who had been up and already had gone out for exercise!

Olga was not the pilgrim for whom we had to wait; in fact, Olga was the one leading and encouraging us. She was willing to share with the others on the pilgrimage her daily exercise regime "to keep you limber", she said. As some members of our group, many years her junior, were dealing with the aches and pains associated with old age, Olga had advice for all of them!

Olga. Some call her "The Magnificent" and indeed she is an inspiration to me. Her zeal for life, her deep faith in God, and her dedication to her family, church, community, and the sports world are why it is not an exaggeration to refer to her as MAGNIFICENT.

Most Reverend Ken Nowakowski
Bishop of New Westminster for Ukrainian
Catholics in British Columbia & Yukon

It was August 2009 at the World Masters outdoor track and field championships in Lahti, Finland; I had travelled back to my homeland to cheer my dad on as he competed in the grueling marathon at these championships for the first time. The excitement surrounding this competition and the athletes rivaled that of any Olympics—but the buzz was all about this 90-something-year old Canadian phenom who had been breaking all kinds of records in both track and field events.

Throwing the javelin twice as far as the second-place competitor in her age group, running 5 seconds faster in a 100-meter sprint, jumping heights rivaling women 10 years her junior. Her name was Olga Kotelko, and I knew I had to meet her.

I'm not entirely sure what I pictured Olga to look like or be like given her performances and star-like prominence at this track meet. Petite yet strong, humble yet confident were my immediate impressions, and being an exercise physiology professor and researcher at McGill University, I marveled at how she was able to accomplish what she had: 11 gold medals in 11 events over an 8-day period, not to mention that 8 of those events were world records!

I invited Olga to visit our research laboratory in the Department of Kinesiology at McGill, so that we could study the limits of her physiological capacity. Without hesitation, Olga agreed (but only after she finished her European cruise), and in March 2010, we put Olga through a battery of tests: measuring her peak capacity to utilize oxygen during exercise, taking a small biopsy of her thigh muscle to investigate under the microscope, testing her maximal muscle strength. This assessment was notably memorable as we brought Olga to the fitness center where she was surrounded by 20-something year old male students who abruptly stopped doing their workout to watch in amazement as a 91-year old woman proceeded to bench-press 60 pounds, a feat that I, more than half her age, could not do!

Simply put, Olga is inspirational—to so many people and in so many ways. She has inspired my husband, Russ Hepple (professor and scientist also at McGill), and me to expand our initial physiological study on Olga to include a larger group of world-class Masters athletes over the age of 75, with the aim of trying to understand how they maintain such superior physiological and cognitive functioning. Olga has inspired numerous young minds here at the university who have seen her undergo testing in the research lab and who have seen her guest lecture in my classes about her training practice and philosophy. In a larger sense, Olga inspires anyone she comes in contact with across the age span to be physically active and to believe in themselves. I'm not sure if we'll ever discover Olga's secret to success, but the experience of knowing her has enriched my life forever. If you can't meet Olga personally, this book is the next best thing!

Dr. Tanja Taivassalo
McGill University Associate Professor
Department of Kinesiology and Physical Education

I first met Olga when she had just begun her track and field career at age 77. Now at the age of 94 her athletic achievements continue to impress me and many others. In the words of Olga's first coach, Bob Robinson, "This super-senior has achieved more in the realm of senior female track and field athletics than any other Canadian and indeed more than any athlete in her age in the whole world".

The spirit of the true athlete does not simply show in competition but in practice as well. Olga has embraced athletics as a second career. She maintains a positive disposition that makes it extremely easy for coaches to work with her. She is extremely dedicated, persevering through a constant program of exercise, which includes general and functional weight training and cardio training in addition to her track and field technical training.

Olga recently returned from the 2012 World Masters Indoor Competition in Jyvaskyla, Finland with a cache of 10 gold medals. There were only 3 competitors in her age category, but the truth is that she smashed world records and at her age is still improving on her past performances.

Olga's message to seniors is that life can be beautiful no matter what your age. Listen to your body and get moving. Aging may be affected by our genes, but our real biological age depends largely on our daily habits, stress level and mental and physical exercise. Her book *Olga: The O.K. Way to a Healthy, Happy Life* will provide readers with inspiration as well as her personal program and strategy for achieving that success.

Barb Vida
Athletic Coach & Personal Trainer

———————

Olga Kotelko is an athlete who excels in a number of track and field events, winning medals and beating the competition in contests all over the world. She can also bench press weights that would challenge any man. One other thing: Olga is 92 years old.

She has the physique, the strength, and the stamina of someone 20 or more years younger. Olga is so extraordinary that scientists who study the mystery of aging are trying to unlock the secret of her longevity.

Saying Olga Kotelko is aging well is a little like saying Wayne Gretzky was pretty good with the puck.

The track and field star owns 27 world records, has won more than 650 medals. If you go to a Masters World Championship anywhere on the planet, people will know who Olga Kotelko is. Research into aging is a relatively new field of study. Until 20 years ago most researchers thought turning back the aging clock was impossible. Aging may be inevitable, but more and more scientists believe how we age can be changed.

From the documentary portrait of *Olga the Magnificent*
CBC Radio, Sunday December 4, 2011

———————————

Because we keep going, and going, and going . . .
Aren't old folks supposed to park their walkers in front of TV sets and slot machines? Dal Richards (93) still leads his big band; Gordon Smith (92) paints as brilliantly as ever; Olga Kotelko (92) holds all 17 world track-and-field records for her age class; Cornelia Oberlander (86) remains a landscape architect of renown; Jimmy Pattison (82) operates one of the largest private companies in Canada. Hey, David Suzuki: great that you've launched a new TV show, but we'll be more impressed when you do it again 10 years from now when you're 85.

Vancouver Magazine, June 2011

———————————

"It is not so much the fear of dying that disturbs me but the sudden awareness that I have just begun to live."

Christopher Plummer
Canadian actor who at the age of 82
was the oldest actor to win an Academy Award in 2012

One
Hitting the Sports Radar at 75

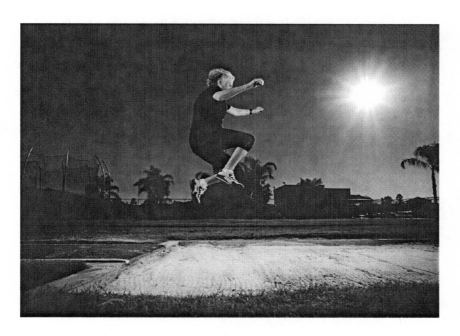

Photo of my long jump at Citrus University, Los Angeles, California, 2010, that accompanied *The New York Times* article, "The Incredible Flying Nonagenarian". Patrik Giardino photo.

In 1994, while playing on a North Shore slo-pitch team, I showed up on the sports radar when I made a double play putting out runners at 1st base and home plate. It was a very good play, yet I think it was because I was a 75-year-old grandmother that people sat up and took notice of me. Aren't little old ladies supposed to be sitting in front of their TVs knitting?

For a number of years, I loved playing the game of slo-pitch, but I decided to give my place to someone younger. I was determined, however, to stay active, so I had to find another fun but challenging physical activity. Two West Vancouver physical education teachers introduced me to track and field competition, and I embraced it with a passion I had not felt for a long time. How does someone start competing in track and field at 77 years of age?

Reporters soon started calling me for interviews: I heard from publications as diverse as *The North Shore News*, *The Saskatoon Star Phoenix*, *The Register-Guard City* in Eugene Oregon, *Reader's Digest*, *Zoomer* magazine, France's *Le Monde*, and *Stella* magazine.

Bruce Grierson, a Vancouver writer who was writing a book on super-agers, accompanied me to Montreal, where I was invited to take part in a McGill University research project. The scientists hoped to determine whether it was my genes or my training that contributed to my strength and stamina. Bruce documented the entire experience and submitted his article to *The New York Times*, where it appeared in November 2010 as their magazine's cover story entitled, "The Incredible Flying Nonagenarian". My computer literate friends told me I had "gone viral".

Numerous local, national, and international radio and television programs, such as CBC's *As It Happens*, *The National* with Peter Mansbridge, BC's *Global News*, and the BBC have interviewed me. In anticipation of the World Cup Soccer 2014 and the 2016

Summer Olympics in Brazil, a Brazilian television crew flew to Vancouver, and they spent an entire weekend watching me train, even attending the St. Mary's church fall bazaar, where they became acquainted with my Ukrainian customs.

When I turned 90, a member of the Canadian Masters Athletic Association introduced me as the *Queen Mother* of multiple events athletes. What a privilege! Yes, I am truly honoured that people celebrate my athletic accomplishments. It's true that I'm the only woman over 90 who is still jumping at masters track and field championships. Physiologists have checked my muscles and found no indication of age-related weakness. Many people are curious to know how and why I seem to be aging so well, and I'm not surprised. The quest for a magic elixir, the Fountain of Youth, is timeless. Since ancient times, people have been looking for the secret to live longer and maintain their youthful vim and vigour.

Over the years, friends and strangers alike have remarked on my good health: "Olga," they say, "you continue to scale mountains and arrive successfully on the other side. Others find it hard to match your energy and passion." I always tell them the same thing: It is never too late to feel good and healthy all over. If I can do it, you can too! I'm really not that special.

If people ask who I am, this is what I reply: Throughout the years, I have been a daughter, a sister, a wife, and a friend. I was a school teacher for 34 years, and a traveller most of my life. Today, I'm a mother, a grandmother, an aunt, a friend, and an athlete.

As we age, we grow into a new version of ourselves; we take on a new identity, perhaps through necessity and perhaps through choice. After awhile, in some cases, through circumstances, we leave that version of ourselves behind. That's part of life. In my lifetime, I have welcomed the chance to grow and become a more mature

Olga because with each new version of myself I gained the confidence to experience life and meet its challenges.

As a teacher I was fortunate to choose a lifelong career for which I was well suited—intellectually, emotionally, and physically. As someone wisely said, it's easy to do what needs to be done, but oftentimes it's hard to discover what you truly love to do.

I am also a fierce competitor by nature, perhaps too fierce. At one of my last international competitions, I met a fellow athlete who has competed against me in the same age category for years. I noticed that on this trip she was accompanied by a caregiver. Could it possibly be her last international competition? Was it the last time I would be competing against her? Today I ask myself: why didn't I let her win at least one gold medal? Why did I take all 11 gold medals in the events in which we competed? A friend suggested that I should simply mail the team member a gold medal. No, that won't do. I should have let her win one gold medal, but would that be fair and square? She, too, was a competitor. Would she have wanted me to *let* her win?

I am a warrior, not a worrier, and I don't do guilt. I'm an optimist who moves forward with focus and determination. I'm not one of those people who believes the past is better than the present. I don't do nostalgia. Everything from our past eventually fades away after it serves its purpose. I have discovered that life is meant to be an adventure, and I haven't come to the end yet!

Over the years, many people have asked me to share my exercise and nutrition strategies, and I have given motivational talks to many people both young and old. Recently, I was encouraged to share my exercise regime, nutrition program, and personal stories in a book and, after giving it some thought, I agreed. While I was writing down my thoughts and recollections, I found my heart was filled with many emotions. As with many people, I have experienced my fair share of sadness and stress, and I found ways to overcome these hardships that I wish to share with you. Adversity can hit all of us. Everyone has hurdles in life, their personal ups and downs. There is no training program, no nutritional secret that makes us immune to misfortune and hardship. It's been said that stories also have the power to inspire and to heal, and I believe they do.

As a teacher, nothing gave me greater pleasure than to observe the look of comprehension that came over my students' faces when I saw that they had learned an important lesson, something of value that may benefit them for the rest of their lives. What I have learned and experienced over my long life may help you to achieve the same physical, mental, and spiritual benefits I enjoy. This is not a memoir; I didn't want to stay trapped in never-ending nostalgia. I want people who read my story to believe that it is possible to embark on the road to health—one firm step at a time—by starting to move in the direction of well-being. Exercise has been my salvation. For instance, we know regular walking and swimming are low impact aerobic exercises. These are excellent exercises to keep our muscles strong, active, and balanced.

To ensure that you benefit from reading my story, I have crafted each of the chapters in my book as a lesson to be learned. I've assigned homework, so be prepared. No cheating! I hope that you will do the work. It's the OK way to a happy and healthy body, mind, and spirit. I may be skilled at throwing weapons such as javelins, hammers and, discus but, as a school teacher I know that education is the most powerful weapon you can use to change the world.

Just for fun, I end each chapter with some of my favourite jokes. A day without laughter is like a day without sunshine. American humorist Mark Twain believed: "Age is a state of mind over matter. If you don't mind, it doesn't matter," and comedienne Lucille Ball said, "The secret of staying young is to live honestly, eat slowly and lie about your age!" Age is just a number.

Longevity is increasing, so plan to spend your days as happy, healthy days. Live, love, laugh, and learn!

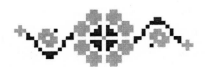

Artwork adapted from designs along the Danube by Olga Kotelko.

At one point during a game, the coach said to one of his young players, "Do you understand what cooperation is? What a team is?"

The little boy nodded.

"Do you understand what matters is whether we win together as a team?" The little boy nodded.

"So," the coach continued, "when a strike is called or you're out at first, you don't argue or curse or attack the umpire. Do you understand that?"

Again the little boy nodded.

"Good! Now go over and explain that to your mother."

Two
My Early Years

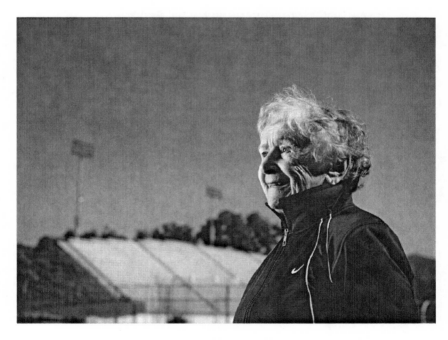

A friendly chat with photographer Patrik on the
track in LA 2010. Patrik Giardino photo.

Lesson: A happy, healthy family is one of the basic building blocks in a healthy community. Next to our life's work, our close personal relationships are extremely important in forming who we were, who we are, and who we will become. The values I learned on the family farm have guided me in life, in particular the value of hard work.

"Don't judge each day by the harvest you reap but by the seeds you plant."
— *Robert Louis Stevenson*

I never imagined when growing up on the family farm in Smuts, Saskatchewan that I would be doing what I am doing today. The road from the family farm to world class athletics was a long and arduous one, and it seems that I had begun to challenge gravity even as an infant.

I was born on March 2, 1919 to Wasyl Shawaga and Anna Bayda, the seventh of their eleven children. As was the custom at six weeks of age, I was taken to be baptized at St. John the Baptist, our Ukrainian Catholic church. My father had hitched up a team of horses to the family sleigh, and while mother and my then six brothers and sisters snuggled under down-filled quilts, laughing and talking about the upcoming special occasion, I was bundled up and sleeping peacefully in the sleigh.

With only a few miles to go, mother checked on me. No baby Frances! The baby wasn't there! They found me about a mile back, sleeping on the snow, still snug in my blanket. There was no back-board on the sleigh, and I guess I had gradually worked my way to the back of the sleigh, slid out, and landed right side up. I really don't remember! Nor do I remember the baptismal ceremony, but the day was significant because for the first, but not the last time in my life, an external event contributed to the formation of my identity. In this case, the priest disapproved of 'Frances', the name my parents had chosen to call me. He preferred 'Olga', so Olga I became, and that has been my name ever since.

My mother's father, Michaylo Bayda (1855–1937), was the eldest son of Fedko Bayda (1831–1883) and Maria Yakowich. My maternal grandfather was born near the village of Zabokroku, in the county of Horodenka, Province of Halychena, Ukraine. He later became a policeman in that area.

Michaylo and his 40-year-old wife Maria left their homeland and immigrated to Canada in 1901. They arrived with the hope of gaining independence, security, and freedom, and the goal of preserving their beliefs, culture, and traditions.

In preparation for a Shawaga family reunion 1901–1986, my sister Phyllis researched our ancestry. She discovered that a branch of the family, our maternal DNA that stretched beyond Michaylo, might be associated with a Ukrainian nobleman. My mother's family, the Baydas, may have descended from Prince Dmytro Bayda Vishnevetsky (1516–1563). Since we don't have definitive proof, for instance a sample of DNA, it is impossible to confirm that association. Yet when I look at my belief that life is an adventure, and recognize that I am both a fierce competitor and a warrior, it just might be true. Cultural genetics, if you like, can also act as an external force in the construction of one's character. The Prince may have been influential in the formation of my identity and contributed to my athletic success.

Prince Vishnevetsky, who lived in Ukraine during the reign of Ivan the Terrible, was a descendant of the Lithuanian Prince

Olgerd, a renowned leader in the colourful history of Ukrainian Cossacks. Cossacks were groups of East Slavic and Turk, or mixed-origin people, who originally were members of democratic, semi-military communities in different regions of Ukraine and Southern Russia from the era of Genghis Khan and the Mongol Hordes. The word "Cossack" denotes a privileged position. It is of Turkish origin, meaning "free man", "guard", "escort", and "adventurer". Perhaps my adventurous spirit comes from these ancient links.

Cossacks were mainly made up of serfs who preferred the dangerous freedom of the wild steppes rather than life under the harsh rule of cruel nobility. The Cossacks who lived on the steppes of Ukraine were notorious, and their numbers increased greatly between the 15th and 17th centuries. Usually they were led by princes, merchants, or runaway peasants from the area of the Poland-Lithuanian Commonwealth. Cossack society was ethnically diverse, and some Cossacks may have had their origins from as far away as Scotland. Jews also served in the ranks of the Cossacks. The Zaporozhians were the most famous among the Cossacks, and they were generally indifferent to religious matters. If you were brave and craved freedom they welcomed you.

Prince Vishnevetsky came from an area in southern Ukraine called Volyn Hedyminovychiv. He was the owner of landed estates in the Kremenets district. In the three year period between 1550–1553, he was mayor of Cherkassy and Kanevsky counties. Around 1552 he built on the island Khortytsya a small castle, which became the prototype of the Zaporizhzhya Sich, the fortified capital located on the Dnieper River and the home of the legendary Cossacks. Since Cossacks were major characters in Ukrainian folklore, the Zaporozhians, in particular, were renowned for their heroic raids against the Ottoman Empire.

In October 1557, Prince Vishnevetsky led 600 Cossack horsemen to free several thousand Ukrainian slaves being held by the Turks. The Turks could be unbelievably cruel to their Ukrainian captives. For example, they would blind oarsmen to prevent their escape from the slave ships. Fortunately, the Prince and his men successfully captured the Turkish fortress and freed the slaves.

Slavery was such an important part of Ottoman society. So many Slavs were enslaved for centuries that the very name 'slave' is derived from the Slavic people, not only in English but in other European languages. Eight years after he captured the Turkish fortress, in early 1563 during a campaign to Moldova, Prince Vishnevetsky was captured and was sent to Constantinople. The heroism and martyrdom of the prince were celebrated in the national parliament, or Duma.

Prior to their defeat, the Turkish leader demanded that the Cossacks submit to Turkish rule. A famous picture by Ilya Repin (1844–1930) entitled *The Reply of the Zaporozhian Cossacks to the Sultan of Turkey* hangs today in the State Russian Museum in St Petersburg. This painting depicts the gathering of Zaporozhian Cossacks as they pen a reply to the Turkish sultan. Their apparent glee suggests they were deriving great pleasure in composing insults to hurl at their enemy.

The artist Repin greatly admired the Cossacks, saying, "All that Gogol wrote about them is true! A holy people! No one in the world held so deeply freedom, equality and fraternity."

Understandably, the battlefield presented opportunities for past generations of Ukrainians to experience victories and defeats, but I prefer the less violent arena of track and field to celebrate freedom, equality, fraternity, and sisterhood.

Fast forward several centuries.

Back in 1901 at the start of the 20th century, the Bayda family—Michaylo, Maria and their children, Nicola (20), Maria (17), Fedor (15), my mother Anna(12) and Iwan (7)—arrived in Canada after sailing from Hamburg, Germany, across the Atlantic Ocean. The family arrived in Halifax, Nova Scotia on May 31, at 6 p.m. (Their son Dmytro would be born in Canada.)

My maternal grandparents and their five children left Halifax and travelled by train via Winnipeg, Manitoba to Rosthern, Saskatchewan where Michaylo's brother, Andree met them. He and his wife Paraska Slusar and family had immigrated to Canada in 1899 and had homesteaded in the Alvena district. Michaylo applied for and was granted a homestead in July, 1901. Their first home was a hovel, a miserable dwelling on the side of a bank of earth. The two parents and their children, aged twenty to seven, lived together in this cramped space. My mother Anna was twelve years old at the time. Later my grandfather erected a log house where Anna lived until she married my father, Wasyl Shawaga.

My father's parents, Stephan Shawaga and Anastazia Konowaluk, came from the village of Harasymiw in the county of Horodska, in Halychyna, Ukraine. My grandfather Stephan was born June 8, 1854, and my grandmother Anastazia was born July 12, 1864. They had six children: Dmytro (1883), my father Wasyl (1887), Mike (1890) and Jim (1895), all born in Ukraine; in Canada, Nastia was born in 1902, and Nick was born in 1905.

The Dominion Lands Act passed in 1872 allowed a settler to a quarter section of unoccupied Dominion land as a homestead for the payment of $10.00 registration fee. After three years, the settler might file a claim of ownership if he could show proof that he had broken a specific number of acres and had built a residence on it.

In the spring of 1905, teenage Wasyl filed for homestead rights for 160 acres in the SW ¼ of Section 28, Township 40, Range 1, West of the 3rd Meridian. He cleared and broke 2 acres and raised a crop by fall. It was only then that he asked my mother Anna to marry him. Anna had caught his eye when both families first met onboard the steamship *Bulgaria* during the long voyage across the Atlantic. Their ship, which carried 717 passengers, was not a fancy cruise ship, but a sturdy basic boat with livestock as well as people. The two families sailed on this ship and settled in their own respective homesteads eight miles apart in the same community.

Father and mother would settle in a small hamlet called Smuts, ten miles outside of Vonda, northeast of Saskatoon. My father was 19 and my mother 17 when they married on November 26, 1906. That year, Wasyl broke another 3 acres and cropped 3 more acres by fall. He also acquired 10 head of cattle and 2 pigs. By 1909 Wasyl and Anna broke and cropped many more acres. The clearing of the land was all hand labour. The land was stoney, and the stones had to be picked by hand. Oxen were then used to plough the land.

By 1910, Wasyl owned 9 head of cattle, 3 horses and 4 pigs. He had built a 16' x 24' log house at a cost of $150. He built an 18' x 30' log barn at a cost of $30, a 16'x 26' granary for $100, and had dug a well at a cost of $20.

Like many who left small plots in the homeland, these early Ukrainian settlers were overjoyed to farm hundreds of acres of land. This made any hardship they endured worthwhile. My father was ambitious, and he was determined to be a good farmer. Eventually he would own 16 farms (quarters).

My parents were compassionate and loving people but had little, if any, formal education. Everything they accomplished was done through practical intuition—how they started their married life together and how they carried on from there. They trusted that if they adhered to fundamental values, their hard work would lead them toward a prosperous future. Despite their lack of formal education, my parents taught us integrity and an unflappable work ethic. Father believed in duty, order, respect, and commitment to a goal: he taught me that with effort anything was possible. You just had to think your way through it.

My mother not only cared for the family but, like many other farm wives, she also helped her husband with the land work. She would hitch two oxen and one horse to a plough while father used five horses to work the land. In 1919, they built a large modern 6 room, two storey house on the property. On March 2nd of that year I was born in our new house. As testament to their skill, the house is still standing.

My parents lived by the sweat of their brow and enjoyed the fruit of their labour. Everything they needed and wanted was grown, built, or baked. Their marriage was an example of beautiful teamwork, and I was fortunate to witness what a successful marriage can look like.

Smuts was a small farming community with few amenities besides the two large grain elevators, a grocery store, and the Ukrainian Catholic church—St. John the Baptist—that our family attended every Sunday. The main roads were built using a steamer engine, while side roads were built with road gangs composed of farmers who worked for the county to pay their taxes. By 1927, father travelled those thoroughfares in his new Model T Ford.

Both of my parents took great interest in their community and both worked devoutly for the Catholic Church, where father served on the parish executive for many years. He was one of the founding members who helped build the church. He also served on the executive of the Riel Dana School, a rural one-room schoolhouse, where as many as 47 pupils attended.

Compared to Smuts, Vonda was a bustling little town. Father would visit there often, and he made friends easily with many people in town: the doctor, the lawyer, the grocer, the blacksmith. Father was a good networker. He learned to read and speak English fluently from his English friends. His philosophy in life and in business was to strive for excellence—Be bold, be you, but most of all, be true to who you are.

Mother would have a baby every two years, so she was kept busy. She would give birth to eleven children: five sons and six daughters. I was near the middle: Mike, Mary, Ann, Jean, John, Matt, Olga, Steve, Phyllis, Kay, and Alex. Besides human babies, the farm produced quite a few other young. My brother Mike remembered that one spring when all the animals were grazing, he counted 51 new births on the farm: colts, calves, piglets, kittens, and puppies.

Jean remembered that mother loved to sing, and although she never learned to speak English as well as father, she had little jingles for every occasion. Phyllis heard mother recite "Twinkle, twinkle, little star," and asked mother where she had learned it. Mother replied she learned it from Mike when he went to school. She recited it beautifully.

> *Tweenkle, tweenkle littiw star,*
> *How woo wunder what yu are*
> *Up above the noisey high*
> *Like ai diamon in a sky.*

Mother was a pillar in our small farming community, and she was respected for her care and consideration. During the deadly flu epidemic of 1918 when many children and neighbours were sick and dying, mother left her own family and young children to make the rounds of the community to offer her help. Eventually, she contracted the flu herself and was sick for three weeks. I recall someone told me all of her children had to spit into a cup, and mother ingested this unusual microbe-rich concoction. We'll never know if it was that strange brew or her tenacity and determination to survive that contributed to her healing but, thankfully, mother recovered from the deadly flu and continued to enjoy her large family.

Farm women were self-reliant. Mother sewed all of our clothes, and she knitted sweaters, mitts and scarves. She raised geese for food as well as for the feathers that were used to make pillows and quilts. Together with her daughters she milked as many as 15 cows by hand. She sold butter and cream, which paid for necessities, and made her own soap for the laundry.

As the family grew, each spring mother planted not one but two huge gardens. My sister said it was "as big as half of Saskatchewan"; everything we ate came from the farm. Today everyone wants to eat locally grown organic food. When I was growing up everything we ate was organic. Chemicals did not appear on the farm until after the Second World War. Father made sure we had a warm house and enough to eat, but there were few treats. I remember vividly one time he brought home a box of apples, and another time a big box of ripe, red tomatoes. We didn't plant tomatoes in our garden at that time, so we learned how to eat and enjoy tomatoes!

During harvest time, neighbour would help neighbour. In the morning, as many as eight men left their own farms to start working in our fields. At 10 a.m., we brought lunch for those hard-working people. By noon, we called them to come to the house where mother would have prepared a banquet of wholesome nourishing foods like borscht, homemade chicken noodle soup, creamed dill potatoes, pyrogies, cabbage rolls, roast beef, and pork.

Eventually, over the years, farmers became more self-sufficient. They bought more machinery and more land and worked only for themselves. Father was good at seeing opportunities. With 11 children you had better be! He was one of the first farmers to go to the local native Indian reserve for help. He became friendly with some of the unemployed young men. These native men would come every summer to help father on the fields, since by then my older brothers and sisters had left home.

Although I was only two years old at the time, I was often told the following story. One spring day, a federal census agent drove to our farm and interviewed father. Dad was preoccupied with the upcoming work to be done, and I think he was distracted as he rattled off the names of his children. He forgot my name! The repercussions of omitting me became evident only later in my life. Although I had a baptismal record, I was never able to get an official birth certificate, and I had problems proving who I was until I received a Certificate of Canadian Citizenship when I attended Normal School in Saskatoon for teacher training. Once again, I had to deal with an issue of my identity: in legal terms, I didn't even exist until I gained the title of teacher. Thank goodness I had found a way to breathe life into my physical self.

It is easy to understand my father's preoccupation with the farm. There always was so much work to be done. From sunrise to sunset we all pitched in to do our share of work on the farm. Before going off to school, we milked 15 cows by hand, separated the cream from the milk, and washed breakfast dishes for 15 people—our immediate family and two hired hands.

In 1926, father bought a Case tractor and a Waterloo threshing machine in partnership with Peter Stadnyk. They worked together for three years until father bought his own outfit. During harvest time, my older brothers and sisters would help father bring in the grain. Four horses pulled the binder and, after the wheat was cut, the sheaves were "stooked" or stacked upright to dry before going to the rack. From the rack, the sheaves of wheat were pitched onto a conveyor belt where they would go through the threshing machine. The grain would be loaded into the wagon to go to the granary, and the straw would be blown to the other side to be used for the animals.

Father was never sick, but he did suffer a few accidents during his farming career that required hospitalization. Once in the fall, while he was hauling a load of wheat to the Vonda elevator, he was walking beside his horses to keep warm and slipped under the wagon and suffered a broken leg. Another time, he was caught between the horses and the seed drill and suffered a few broken ribs. When he was cutting chaff for his stock with his sons, his clothing got caught in the rotating shaft, which threw him over and dislocated many joints in his hands and feet.

After all of their children had married and moved out on their own, father and mother gave up farming and moved to Saskatoon for a well-deserved rest. They bought a little house on 22nd Street, close to the church, and moved into the city house in the fall of 1953.

One day I encouraged my mom and dad to take a professional photograph in a studio in Saskatoon. There they were, perched on a piano bench, my dad straddling the bench, sweating profusely in the dark suit he seldom wore. Mom looked lovely with her long, brown hair pinned into tight curls. As I look at their photo today, I realize how young she looked for her years, despite all the hard work.

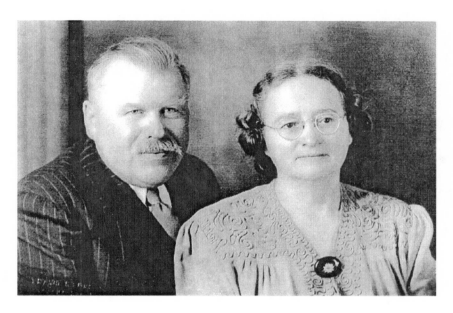

My parents, Wasyl and Anna Shawaga.

Mother said the only time in her life she had seen our father cry was at the last Christmas they spent on the farm. Although they had eleven children and numerous grandchildren, not one family member had thought to go out to the farm to spend Christmas with them. It was the first time our parents celebrated the Christmas holiday alone.

My parents were kind, helpful, and respectful people, both morally and financially. They demonstrated a steadfastness of purpose that inspires me to this day. They lived together for 55 years, celebrating their 50th anniversary in 1956. After a short illness, Wasyl died on Sunday August 6th, 1961 at the age of 74. Anna died on Sunday September 22, 1974 at the age of 85. She had planted her own garden in the spring of 1974.

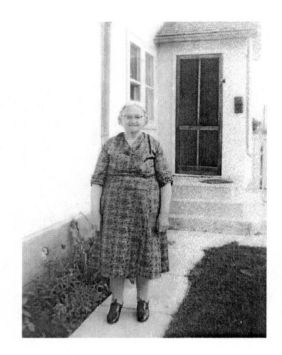

Mother standing in front of her Saskatoon
home a short time before her death.

School!

The story of my experiences at the one-room rural school was one
of initiative, determination, achievement, difficulties, disappoint-
ments and, above all, courage. In March 1924, when I turned five
years old, I entered grade 1 in Riel Dana School, a typical rural
one-room schoolhouse, two miles from our farm. In the summer
we walked to school. In winter, we travelled by horses hitched to
a caboose. The horses were kept in a barn near the school house,
and it was our brother Steve, a lover of horses, who hitched and
unhitched them, and who took us to and from school.

For my first day of school, my older sister, Jean, had made me a burgundy velvet dress embroidered with beads. That dress was the envy of all. Although the idea never entered my head, I think I must have been the cutest kid in the bunch!

Mrs. Savella Stechishin was my grade 1 teacher. I loved her, and I loved my new life. In later years, Mrs. Stechishin enjoyed meeting with me socially, and she always praised me to her friends. I admired this gracious lady, and I believed in her life philosophy. When anyone asked her advice, she humbly said, "My goal always is to be my best, to embrace a healthy lifestyle, and to accept new challenges. Be positive and happy. Be your best today. Do I think older is better? Yes I do!" Mrs. Stechishin passed away recently. She published the famous cookbook, *Traditional Ukrainian Cookery*.

My brothers and sisters and I would rush to finish our farm chores so that we could get to school and play before classes started. Our favorite game was softball, *if* we had a bat and *if* we could find a ball. In some schools, naughty students would take the globe and use it as a ball.

Some teachers would suspend their globes near the ceiling as protection against being 'borrowed'. In other one-room schools, mice enjoyed the glue used to make the globes and would nibble away at foreign lands and sections of ocean.

Although I really wasn't a serious athlete in school, I did like softball. Mary Scherban Lelach and I were the only two girls on the rural school championships baseball team. After school ended at 4 o'clock, we would often walk 6 miles to a neighbouring school, play the ball game, and walk back home sweaty and tired but happy.

Another favorite game was called "Anti, Anti Over". One group of kids would be on one side of the schoolhouse, and another group was positioned anxiously on the other side. Someone would throw the ball over the school roof, and you would try to catch it. Then the opposing side would rush over and try to take a prisoner. The group that had the most prisoners won. It was great fun, and it made you tough.

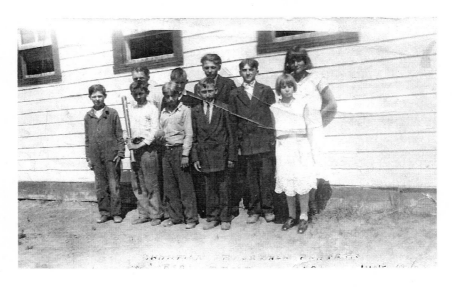

The Rak School softball team in 1931 with me in the first row.

We played hopscotch and marbles as well as skipping rope. At lunch time, we would conjure up pageants and pretend we were at a wedding. Someone played the bride, a groom and, of course, we would need a priest and bridesmaids. We had so little in the way of game equipment and props, or stories from the cinema to model, that we made the most of our imaginations. Remember, this was the era before electricity and television.

I enjoyed school, liked my teachers, and was curious about the stories we read in library books. I learned to read, print, write and, eventually, to type. Little did I know at the time that it would become a valuable asset.

I excelled in every subject—mathematics, history, science, geography, and social studies. I remember one unfortunate incident in a grade 5 math class. Although I was good in math, for whatever reason I was unable to solve a particular problem that the teacher had written on the blackboard. I stood there self-consciously, unable to answer the problem, and feeling quite embarrassed in front of all those staring eyes. As punishment, the teacher put me under his desk.

There I was, crammed under the teacher's desk along with another unfortunate student for the rest of the math class. After school, the teacher lined up the four of us who had had difficulty in math that day and lashed us with a willow branch. When our parents saw all the welts and bruises on our shoulders they were furious, and the teacher was immediately dismissed from our school.

After I completed grades 8, 9, and 10 by correspondence courses, my parents sent me to complete grades 11 and 12 at Saskatoon's Bedford Road Collegiate. I lived with the Sister Servants of Mary Immaculate, an order of Catholic nuns. My parents did not have enough money to pay for my accommodations, so they bartered with the nuns: my father's potatoes and cabbages paid for my room and board.

I must not neglect to add this memory. When living on the farm as a youngster, every summer for two weeks I walked each day with the other children five miles to our parish church. A fledgling community of Sister Servants of Mary Immaculate (SSMI) nuns taught us catechism and religious instructions. They formed in me a faith that I may often take for granted, but will always respect. Their guidelines were founded in the importance of following the precepts of a Christian life. Every individual's talent was developed and valued with respect. I have always believed in and admired their tireless work. I am grateful to have had the SSMI in my life.

Although I loved the sisters, and I once dressed up in a nun's habit just to see how it felt, the thought of entering the religious orders never crossed my mind. I believe I was the only boarder who was not studying to become a nun. But I did love to study, and eventually in 1935 I attended Secretarial Success Business College. I worked for four years before going to Saskatoon Normal School to become a teacher. I graduated in 1941 and began my teaching career. I later attended the University of British Columbia to complete my undergraduate education. At Normal School I added my middle name, Marlene. Later, when I had to sign my initials, it didn't seem right to simply write *OK*.

I studied secretarial subjects, such as typing, shorthand, and penmanship, skills that became useful in later years. During the assembly at Normal School in Saskatoon, Principal C.P. Sealy asked for a volunteer to work in his office. Although I knew I could do it, I was too scared and timid to volunteer, but my friends pushed me to stand up. There I was, shaking like a leaf, my knees knocking together as I stood in front of Mr. Sealy. "Miss Shawaga, spell the word 'ecstasy'." With great concentration, I recited each letter and then plopped down in my seat.

"I want to see you in my office first thing tomorrow morning."

I got the job. I was ecstatic! I thoroughly enjoyed working for my principal that entire year, all because I was able to type and to spell the word "ecstasy".

Your homework assignment:

Remember those family members who have gone before you. They continue to live on in your heart and mind.

Give thanks to your elders and ancestors, those who are known and those who are unknown.

Remain close to the people you love and who love you. Have a positive attitude so that you will feel loved and needed.

It is not too late to start good habits that can flow down to your future generations. Realize that you can enhance your whole life through your positive actions.

May the love and protection of your ancestors keep you happy, healthy, and safe.

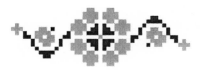

A grandmother was telling her young granddaughter what her own childhood was like: "We used to skate outside on a pond. I had a swing made from a tire; it hung from a tree in our front yard. We rode our pony. We picked wild raspberries in the woods." The little girl was wide-eyed, taking this all in. At last she said, "I sure wish I'd gotten to know you sooner!"

Three
My Teaching Career

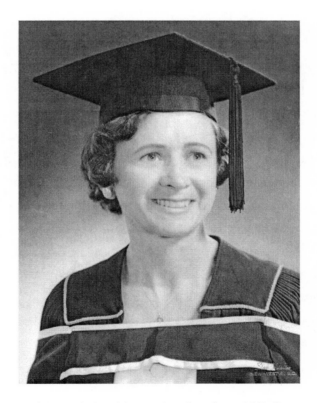

A proud day. My graduation from U.B.C.

Lesson: Each of you possesses an innate talent that demands to be expressed not only for your benefit and for those around you. If you discover those God-given talents and put them to good use, you will discover what brings you joy and happiness in life. Job satisfaction, whether paid or volunteer, provides daily mental challenges and social activity. It takes all kinds of people to make the world.

"By being yourself, you put something wonderful in the world that was not there before."
— *Edwin Elliot*

After graduating as a teacher from Saskatoon Normal School in 1941, I signed a contract with a school trustee in the Rak community for my first teaching position. Men in the community constructed the rural school buildings as close as possible to where families lived. Lands were sometimes donated for this purpose. Communities did the best they could with limited funds. The schools' dimensions were based on standard plans that allowed about fifteen square feet per pupil, approximately ten to eleven-foot ceilings, a window or two, and a mudroom or cloakroom for boots and coats. My classroom, like many others across Saskatchewan, contained shelves for books and lunches, a pot belly stove, students' desks, a teacher's desk and chair, and a blackboard.

The trustees' job was to hire the teacher, buy supplies, guide the running of the school, and meet all sanitary and health conditions. The trustees also had the difficult job of convincing people to pay school taxes, especially those without children to send to school. Most of the trustees had no experience in school management but simply believed in providing an education for the community children.

In those days, many teachers were women because men enlisted in the war, and they did not usually go into the teaching profession. I was hired at a salary of $700 a year; however, if I got married, I would lose my job. Teachers were paid for ten months work and not paid for the summer months of July and August. In my second year of teaching, I earned $900. That year I was able to buy a black seal fur coat for myself. How fashionable I felt.

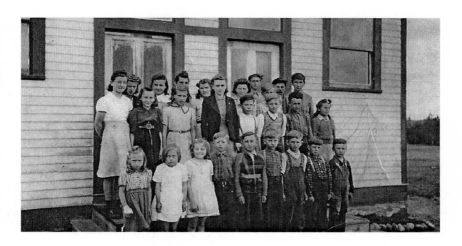

I am the one in the middle wearing a dark jacket
standing with my students in front of our one-room school.

Schools were the center of community life. The schools were used for meetings, social gatherings, dances, and sometimes even as a church. Hallelujah! What fun we had! Parents and neighbours were caring, obliging, and understanding. Everyone was happy and helpful. After the older students completed their assignments, they were eager to volunteer, if needed, to help me with the younger students. All children were obliged to come to school but had to get up early to do chores before going off to school. Some children did not have warm enough clothes to travel the long distances in winter months. Occasionally, new immigrants would arrive unexpectedly. There were never any behavior problems, such as hooky, bullying, or discrimination. Even with the bigger boys, there was never a need for police intervention as one experiences today.

There were eleven subjects on the elementary school timetable: geography, history, music, literature, arithmetic, grammar, written language, nature science, health, art, and citizenship. Good penmanship was stressed. We might have to teach nine grades, and find ourselves staring at students that encompassed a wide range of ages in each grade. For four years in that one-room rural Saskatchewan schoolhouse, I taught grades 1 to 10 and helped grades 8, 9, and 10 with correspondence lessons. Not only did I teach those grades, but I taught *all* subjects to 47 pupils, from the ages of 6 to 17. I felt competent in this particular teaching methodology; it resembled the format in which I had been taught.

Every month I issued report cards to every student in every grade. Each student was rated in all the subjects, and there were never any parental complaints. Many of my students would eventually become teachers, nurses, doctors, lawyers, businessmen and women, and would contribute as great citizens and leaders in their communities. They were tolerant, decent children who came from good, hardy stock. I agree that Canada's future was written on the blackboards of those one-room school houses.

In those days, the students' physical education or gym program was less structured: the daily walks to and from school provided an excellent exercise regime. Nonetheless, my students loved their game of baseball at lunchtime, and they would not play unless I played with them. I was happy to oblige. Although we had limited sports equipment, we learned to be resourceful. I coached them to compete in the community school sports days in Vonda, and we proudly paraded our school banner after winning coloured ribbons and trophies in baseball competitions as well as various races, jumping and throwing events.

Every Friday afternoon we created a program of interesting, funny, or dramatic skits that involved singing and dancing or whatever else was appropriate and suitable entertainment. It was an enjoyable way to end a progressive week until we would meet again on Monday morning. At Christmas we would stage lavish concerts lasting two hours and each and every student was included and would have a role to play.

Besides being the school teacher, I was also the school janitor. It was my responsibility to start the fire in the pot belly stove to heat the schoolroom. I could do that task easily enough, but to fetch water for the children, now that was another story. Obtaining clean water for the schoolhouse was a problem. Although some schools had their own well, potable water was not guaranteed. Sometimes students had to bring their own water from home or fetch it from a nearby creek, river, or other source. Well water could sometimes have a strange taste, smell, or colour and occasionally would be contaminated. A drought brought a huge number of grasshoppers to the prairies. The grasshoppers found their way into schoolhouse wells and into the students' drinking water. The solution was to fit a cotton bag over the water pump's spout. The water, after passing through the cotton bag was clean, but inside the bag was a soggy mess of drowned grasshoppers and other insects.

Some schools arranged for water to be delivered to the school— but not ours. I had to walk across the road to the neighbour's well and carry two heavy buckets of water through knee-high snow, occasionally in 30° below weather. Those buckets of water were heavy and awkward to carry, and it was a long trip. In the winter, the school would be so cold that a layer of ice formed on the top of the water I had brought in. Those are the days that stay in my mind.

On Arbor Day, traditionally a day for beautifying the environment, teachers as well as pupils were obliged to clean the schoolyard. We picked up broken pieces of glass and any other garbage that had accumulated over the year. One spring, we realized that the grass around the school was too tall to rake, so we decided to burn it.

That day, the spring weather was relatively calm with a gentle breeze occasionally blowing from the south. The older students felt quite capable and resilient for the job at hand. Everything went well until a little whirlwind whipped some cinders into larger flames that we could not smother in time. The growing, smoking fire was soon out of control and started to burn a field of stubble on the edge of the neighbour's farm. This was not fun anymore.

We worked furiously, but the fire was getting bigger and bigger as it head for the farmer's yard. Some of us began to pray for help. Suddenly, before we knew it, the fire subsided, changed direction, calmed down, and burnt itself out. A little miracle. We ended that spring day with frazzled nerves but a tidy schoolyard!

Most teachers at that time still had to board with a student's family or with a household looking to make some extra money. Some teachers had to live in granaries, bunkhouses and, in some cases, barns or tents. I was fortunate to reside in the teacherage adjacent to the school, so I did not have to commute daily.

The little teacherage was conveniently located by the school, but was isolated. At night, the coyotes howling on the prairie and the squirrels scurrying up the side of the house kept me company. As a young single female teacher, I occasionally enjoyed the local social scene: the box lunch socials, sweetheart dances, hockey nights, and curling bonspiels. When I arrived back to my living quarters, after a winter evening out with friends, frost glistened on the ceiling, and half-inch hoarfrost icicles clung to every nail on the wall. I will never forget the cold. I want to impress upon you that winters in Saskatchewan could be bitterly cold with the temperature dropping to 30° below and even lower. It was so cold I would layer myself with longjohns, PJs, a hood parka and, occasionally, even mitts. This is how I warmed up in bed. Oh, what memories!

Some of my brothers left school to help father on the farm as there was always plenty of work. A number of them eventually took up farming as an occupation. My sisters married farmers. I always knew that I would marry one day even though I knew it would be the end of my teaching job. I had witnessed my parents' happy and productive marriage and saw that as my goal.

It was love at first sight when I met my husband-to-be, John Kotelko. He was tall, dark, and handsome. He was twenty-six and I was twenty-four. We married in August 1943 in a church on the farm in Cudworth, Saskatchewan. I wore a beautiful long, white dress with a lovely veil that trailed behind me as I walked down the aisle. The whole community of 400 people came out to wish us a happy and prosperous life. A *korovai* is traditional wedding bread that symbolizes community: it takes the place of wedding cake at a Ukrainian reception. Usually, the family and the entire village bake it as an expression of support for the newlyweds: everyone contributes flour to the cake. John and I did not have a *korovai*, but we did have three special breads, or *kolachi*. We did not receive wedding presents, but we did receive \$137.21 as *dorovinya* from the guests, quite a lot of money for 1943.

I remember as John and I were leaving the church after the wedding, a sudden gust of wind blew the veil over my eyes, temporarily blinding me. Perhaps that was an omen. I was blind to how my married life would unfold. I believed in the sacrament of marriage as being an expression of total devotion and commitment to family. I dreamed that my husband and I would love each other for life, just like my parents had done in their marriage. I wished for a lovely family, and was granted this wish when we had two beautiful daughters, Nadine and Lynda but, sadly, the happy family life was not to be. The name 'Kotelko' is believed to have originated from '*kotel*'. In a farm house, a *kotel* is the name for the container that holds hot water within a wood stove. My husband, like his namesake, was prone to over heating when it came to his temper.

John was not a farmer; he worked for an insurance company, which caused him to travel extensively and be away from home for long periods of time. He also preferred activities that took him away from home: he played the fiddle, and often was invited to play at weddings and dances, leaving me at home with Nadine while he went off to enjoy himself. No, he did not stay home and keep me warm. As they grew older, I would warn my two daughters against marrying a man who has to travel for his work.

Truthfully, I was happily married for only the first ten days after the wedding. The image of happily ever after faded quickly when I realized that John had no intention of changing his role from bachelor to husband. Instead, he enjoyed the benefits of cooked meals and a warm bed without contributing to his family's happiness. He would not tolerate any disruption of his routine. He avoided discussions and closed down emotionally. A few days into our marriage, I asked him why he was always so late coming home for dinner. He told me that, as an insurance salesman, his business hours were mainly after supper when the clients would be home from work. He added that if he thought I was sitting at home stewing over his being late, then he would make a point not to hurry. This harsh response gave my blood a chill; this was a side of him I had never seen, and I felt sick. Quickly and dramatically, his lack of interest in his little family made me realize I was on my own, but rather than wallow in pity, I chose to accept his terms and stay out of his way.

He was the master of the house, and controller of the finances. Money was scarce, so I was continually asking for grocery money. He preferred to spend his money socializing with his male friends, so I started a garden and grew vegetables to avoid going hungry and to be more self-sufficient. John wanted a wife, but not the responsibilities that come with marriage, so he and I had no emotional connection with each other. He could be gone from home for as long as a month, and when he returned, Nadine wouldn't recognize him. This was sad, and added to my loneliness. In those days, you didn't consider divorce, especially if you were raised Catholic. I was determined to withstand the challenges, while praying that the situation would improve. Unfortunately, things got worse.

A few years into the marriage, John came home late while I was sleeping. The memory is a bit blurred, but I remember that he woke me up, accusing me of being unfaithful to him. This was not a new accusation, but the incident stood out in my mind because it was the first time he had accused me while holding a butcher knife to my throat. I decided to gather enough strength and courage to leave him. I went to a lawyer and explained that I was worried John might hurt me, and that Nadine could be in danger as well.

The lawyer knew John's character and told me to 'Get the hell out!' At first, I was stumped as to how I could leave without John knowing my plan, but fate intervened in an unfortunate way: his mother had died in her farmyard while feeding the chickens, and we were to go to the funeral. My parents knew of my plan to leave him, and they met us there. I left with them that night, and Nadine and I began a new life, but not for long.

My parents had retired but still lived on the farm. Every morning, Dad would hitch up a team to drive Nadine two miles to school and pick her up in the afternoon. I felt bad watching my parents as they tried to look after us, so I decided to move again. We went to Saskatoon to stay at my Uncle Jim's. This time, Nadine's school was just a short distance away, and we enjoyed the open air skating rink a block from home. We were happy and content without the threat of an angry husband breaking up our peace.

Soon after, I accepted a teaching position in a rural area where Nadine could be one of my pupils. She was six years old and had become my little companion. We were set to leave and had our few boxes packed up. At the train station of our destination, we loaded our few possessions onto a horse-drawn sleigh and rode from the station to the school, excited to be starting a new adventure. When we arrived at the house where we would live, John was waiting for us on the front porch.

My excitement turned to shock then resignation. I understood that my life had taken another wrong turn, and I would have to go with him. Our boots had barely touched the snow, and I hadn't even had a chance to unpack a single box; we got into his car and drove to Canora Saskatchewan where we lived in a hotel. I never learned how he had discovered our whereabouts and would never have questioned him about it.

This time, things were different. One important difference was that I worked as a teacher, so I had my own money. Unfortunately, our living conditions reverted to that earlier unhappiness, but enough time had been spent away from him to give me the will to change our circumstances. I did not want to put Nadine through more distress so, again, I decided to leave him. A new motivation cinched my decision: I was not only worried for Nadine and me, but also for the child I was carrying. I was pregnant and about to travel as far as possible to get away from him, but this time I was better prepared. As my marriage had been unravelling, and I knew major changes were in order, I had started to save money to send to my sister Jean in British Columbia.

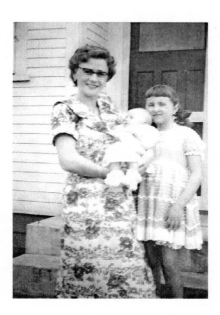

Olga and daughters Nadine and baby Lynda.

Jean was living in New Westminster and had invited us to come west. (Jean was the sister who had made my burgundy velvet dress, embroidered with coloured beads, for my first day in grade one.)

After 10 years of haphazard married life, Nadine was now eight years old and I was pregnant with Lynda. I bid farewell to my beloved Saskatchewan and, in 1953, said hello to beautiful British Columbia. When I arrived, all my sister said was, "What took you so long?"

By the time we arrived in B.C., I had managed to amass almost $1,000. Jean's family, her husband Matt, son Noris, and daughter Adelka lived in New Westminster, and that was where my daughter Lynda was born.

I enrolled Nadine in Lord Tweedsmuir Elementary School in New Westminster, and I went to work in the office of a creosote manufacturing firm. I had received my teacher certificate from Saskatoon Normal School and taught in that province for 4 years. In order to teach in British Columbia, I had to supplement my qualifications with extra hours during the summer as well as night classes, which resulted in my graduating from the University of British Columbia. I began looking for a full-time teaching position as my funds were quickly dwindling. Luckily, within the year, I was hired by the Burnaby School Board.

Within a short time my daughters and I had our own home. I had bought a corner lot in New Westminster for $2,000. Students at New Westminster Senior Secondary High School built a house every year that they sold off as a fundraiser. I was lucky enough to buy a house from them for $5,000 and have it moved to the lot at 2101 Dublin Street. My girls and I loved that home.

I never saw John again. His brother contacted me in 1964 to tell me he had died in Flin Flon, Manitoba. Before we were married, the Air Force had rejected John because he had a collapsed lung. This afflicted him all his life, and his smoking made it worse. Evidently, this was the condition that killed him. He was only forty-seven years old. Out of respect for him and his family, I took his two daughters to his funeral. The three of us slept in his house while his body lay in a closed coffin in the parlour. Once again, we were together under one roof, but this time, I felt safe and calm; my faith helped me to forgive him and to pray for his soul, that I believed was now at peace. He was my children's father, and I never wished him ill will. My daughters and I followed him to the graveside where we said our last goodbyes. That part of our lives was over. My identity as a wife had gradually faded into mother and teacher, two roles I was happy to embrace.

Now that I had obtained the requisite teaching requirements for B.C., I began my new teaching job. I worked with the Burnaby School Board for 30 years, the first 18 in the position of classroom teacher in the elementary grades, and then 12 years as a Hospital and Homebound Teacher before retiring in 1984 at the age of 65.

My teaching career in Burnaby presented me with a slight adjustment in style when compared to my experience in rural Saskatchewan. In the rural schoolroom, I taught all the curriculum subjects to 47 pupils from grades 1 to 10, but at Glenwood Elementary School in B.C., I taught a split class of 18 grade 1 and grade 2 students. I was concerned about handling the situation effectively, so I asked for help from a primary grades' supervisor. She divided each grade into two groups which now seemed like I was teaching four grades. This arrangement made us all happy, however, and we progressed very effectively. Glenwood School was composed of two teaching classrooms, one stacked above the other with two teachers and Mr. Campbell the janitor. Mr. Campbell was such a dear man: he often helped me out by picking up Lynda from St. Peter School in New Westminster and then driving her to my school. A new Glenwood School was being constructed on the property, and in a short while we moved into a new building, and the old school was demolished.

During my 30 years working for the Burnaby School Board, I taught in five schools: Riverway West, Glenwood, Suncrest, Clinton, and Nelson, predominantly in grades 1, 2 and 5. My expertise was the 3R's—reading, writing, and arithmetic as well as art and physical education. For several years, I acted as the Burnaby School District Elementary School art director.

As well as teaching my class, I would give individual help and seminars for teachers during after-school hours. As I write this book, I am reminiscing about my students and the different staff members. I cherish a letter I received from one of these students:

Dear Mrs Kotelko,

About forty-five years ago you made a permanent impression on a little girl. I was in your grade 1 class at Glenwood School, Burnaby. It was my first introduction to being educated and I loved it. "Mrs. Kotelko" challenged her students to always work hard and to do their best. Before the term came into popularity she was a promoter of life-long learning, encouraging her students to love the process of learning, trying new things and improving oneself. As I continued through secondary school to university until I became a teacher myself, I recognized that I had been extremely fortunate to have such a wonderful start to my education.

I lost track of Mrs. Kotelko but I did not forget her. About ten years ago I saw an article in the newspaper. I read that after retirement Olga Kotelko became an athlete and at seventy plus years of age she was in the Seniors Olympics. This was so much like the determined enthusiastic, undaunted woman who sang "Kookaburra" and taught me to read, that I knew it must be "my" Mrs. Kotelko. When I learned that she was giving a workshop at the Vancouver Health and Wellness Show I gathered up my first grade class photos and went downtown to reconnect.

The audience was mostly seniors and as Olga spoke they became engaged in her message of "try something new, challenge mind, body and spirit and see where it takes you". Surrounded by her medals, trophies and awards we were all inspired. There were questions afterwards, some timid, some fearful. With insight, clear directions and lots of humour, Olga answered each one, encouraging and inspiring with her words, her optimism, her "you can do it" approach to sports and to life.

I was not the only student who contacted Mrs Kotelko. Other students called, and this year we had the first Glenwood School Grade 1 reunion dinner. Olga had prepared a package for each of us that came with her words, "You Can Do It". It should be noted that on that evening the actor Harrison Ford was also eating chow mein in the restaurant, but he got very little attention from our table. We had Mrs. Kotelko!

All the newspaper articles, interviews, ribbons and accolades confirm that Olga Kotelko has made overwhelming achievements in the Seniors Olympics and is worthy to be nominated to the Saskatchewan Sports Hall of Fame and Museum. What may not be as evident is that she has always been challenging herself, as a single parent, as a teacher and in her retirement as an athlete. From first grade she inspired her students to find new challenges, do their best and never, ever give up. Forty-seven years later, we all remembered that. Today, Olga Kotelko promotes sports along with her inspiring outlook on life. She is proof and motivation that advancing in age can be a joy and a challenge as much as any other stage in life. At the Aquatic Center in West Vancouver, and the Burnaby Retired Teachers Association, at conferences, on radio and TV, one can always find Olga Kotelko where the action is: full of life, full of laughter, full of new ambitions and goals and full of encouragement for others.

It is a great honour to support her nomination to the Saskatchewan Sports Hall of Fame and Museum.

Caprice Soames August 9, 2005

My Glenwood School students had located their 1958 grade 1 teacher, *Mrs. Kotelko* in 2008. Since we reunited they have been treating me to annual dinners at very fine restaurants. My students are now in their 50s: a businessman, a nurse, a teacher, a firefighter, a horse trainer, and two happily married housewives. It is a delight to relive with them those happy school memories. It reminds me of a lovely quote: "A teacher affects eternity; she/he can never tell where her/his influence stops."

One of my goals as an elementary school teacher was to go beyond teaching my students the 3 R's, and to teach them about life and different cultures. I recall one time when my grade 5 class in Nelson School had completed all of their assignments, were tidying up their desks, and then quietly waiting for the lunch bell. I sat on my desk facing the class and decided to introduce them to my family's Christmas traditions. I shared with them family customs that involved the cooking of special and delicious foods, and explained the intricate preparations that required much effort. I told them that the effort was well worth it because the preparation of the feast created joy and happiness for the whole family. My students learned that for Ukrainians the most beloved and joyful festivity is Christmas.

My students were particularly interested in the Ukrainian foods I prepare for our Christmas Eve meatless supper. The twelve dishes represent the 12 apostles, and include fish soup, borscht, cabbage rolls, and pyrogies. *Kutya* is a dish made of whole wheat cooked for many hours and prepared with honey and poppy seed. The dish symbolizes peace, prosperity, and good health, and everyone around the table must partake of the *kutya* if only but a spoonful.

When the lunch bell rang and the class left for lunch, Kevin ran all the way home, burst through the door and announced to his startled mother, "Mom, Mrs. Kotelko eats the same things we do at Christmas Eve supper!" His mother later related this to me. What precious moments I experienced with my students.

During the last 12 years of my teaching career I was a Hospital and Homebound Teacher. This involved helping students with their lessons and helping them stay connected with their peers while convalescing in the hospital or at home. The advantage of this teaching system was that it was learning on a one-on-one basis. This undoubtedly hastened the student's healing as well.

Sadly, there would also be funerals of very ill students to attend. I vividly remember one student who was determined to excel in math while convalescing from cancer treatments. What a determined young boy! How he loved to do math and how unfortunate was his early death.

Most of the time, I found this work rewarding, especially when a parent would take the time to phone me. One mother said, "What have you done with my daughter Mary? She is so happy to get back to school. You must know how shy and quiet Mary was, and now she is like a new person". I told Mary's mother that I was able to detect Mary's particular weakness in math, and I showed her another way to arrive at the correct answer in a way she was able to understand. "Mary showed me how to teach her," I explained to her mother.

I recall another incident that occurred soon after I started Hospital and Homebound teaching. Doug was 14 years old and doing grade 6 work at home. No school would accept him because of his unruly, undisciplined behaviour. Initially, I had difficulty locating his house that was situated at the back of a weedy, overgrown yard. I walked up the creaking, broken, front steps and knocked at the wood door a couple of times, feeling apprehensive and hesitant but not wanting to give up. The door open slowly, and Doug jumped out from behind the door to startle me. He succeeded! We began with social studies but soon that became tedious for him. We decided to play some number games. A huge dog came to sniff me, and he became rather unpleasant. It was time to leave. I could not get out of the ramshackle house and back to my car fast enough. Back in the office, I broke down in tears in front of my supervisor: "Never again am I going to work with Doug," I exclaimed, hardly able to contain myself.

My years as a Hospital and Homebound Teacher taught me a valuable lesson that I still treasure to this day: It takes all kinds of people to make the world. I learned to put into practice more compassion, devotion, and humility and to take the time to talk to people. I believe one becomes a more resilient person learning through unfamiliar experiences.

"A loving silence often has more power to heal and to connect than the most well intentioned words."
— *Rachel Naomi Remen*

During my 34 years of teaching elementary school I would become addicted to helping people satisfy their innate curiosity. I cherished the years when I witnessed their joy in achieving, through hard work and perseverance, the personal growth needed to become good citizens and respected contributors to society. I feel privileged to have had such an effect on those young minds.

Your homework assignment:

Make a new friend today. A new friend can boost your happiness levels. Renewing a relationship or starting a new one can herald a brand new beginning.

Is there someone from your past, a family member or a friend you've wanted to contact but haven't made time for? Search out a forgotten friend.

If someone has hurt you, today forgive them. Forego a grudge. Apologize if you were wrong.

How are you feeling about your life right now? Do you know what you love to do? What are your talents? Talent usually comes easily and naturally. It's never too late to discover.

Do you find your job satisfying? If not, why not? Is it time for you to retire? Being of service to society is important. Volunteers make the world go round, and there are so many worthy organizations that could use your help. Whether it's teaching, consoling, cooking, painting or singing, share your gifts. Share the great camaraderie. You have more to give than you realize. Work hard, play fair and have fun.

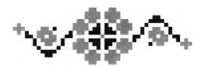

A kindergarten teacher was observing her classroom of children while they were drawing. She would occasionally walk around to see each child's work. As she got to one little girl who was working diligently, she asked what the drawing was. The girl replied, "I'm drawing God."

The teacher paused and said, "But no one knows what God looks like." Without missing a beat, or looking up from her drawing, the girl replied, "You will in a minute."

Four
Travels and Adventures

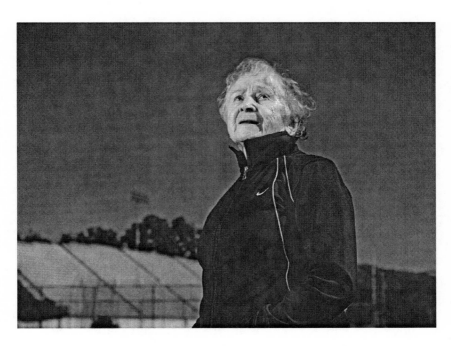

Wishful thinking, travelling to faraway places.
Sailing around the world 1966–1967. Patrik Giardino photo.

Lesson: A wise person said, "If a man or woman has anything in him or her, travel will bring it out, especially ocean travel." Travelling is fun; it broadens the mind. When we are young we travel to discover the world; afterwards, we travel to make sure it is still there. Take pleasure in the beauty and wonder of the world.

My working life was busy and full. For ten months of the school year, I taught my students. For the remaining two months, during the summer, I worked as a lab technician at the Royal City Cannery. After teaching in Burnaby for a number of years, I was offered an exciting opportunity to go on a Teacher Exchange to Nuneaton, England for the 1966–1967 school year. Instead of flying to England in the summer of 1966, my then 13-year-old daughter Lynda and I ventured to sail from Vancouver. I sold my car, a Chevrolet Impala, and with the money bought our tickets. We would circumnavigate the world by cruise ship, leaving from Vancouver in July 1966, travelling via the Orient and the Suez Canal to arrive in Southampton, England in August 1966. Our return from Southampton, at the end of August 1967, took us to Vancouver via the Panama Canal, just in time to resume teaching at Burnaby Suncrest School.

We spent five weeks on the ocean liner *Iberia*, a beautiful ship that was a far cry from the humble boat that brought my parents to Canada. This monster ship contained a crew of 672 and 1384 passengers, of which 651 were in first class. Lynda and I joined the 733 passengers in the tourist/economy class that comprised mainly families with children, making the ship's atmosphere busy, happy, and congenial.

Immediately upon our departure in Vancouver on July 1st, we began the exploration of our vessel as it made its voyage across the calm Pacific Ocean to Hawaii. Our cabin consisted of two double-decker bunks for sleeping and not much room for anything else. We were content with the tiny space as we preoccupied ourselves with the many on-board adventures. Daily activities kept everybody busy and entertained. The children in first class soon realized what a jolly bunch we were in tourist/economy, and they joined us in games.

During this sea voyage, I was no longer 'teacher'. I was a mother and a traveller, two parts of my identity that I loved.

After five days on the Pacific Ocean, we reached the warm shores of Hawaii. After disembarking, we took a day tour of the Island of Oahu. It was a treat to have our feet on solid ground again, if only for the day. In another five days we reached Yokohama, Japan and were greeted on shore by Miss Yokohama. We arranged a three-day overland tour from Yokohama to Kobe via Tokyo and Osaka, visiting many interesting sites. As it was the height of summer, we met numerous groups of youngsters at various exhibitions and tourist sites. Each time we met these black-haired youngsters, neatly dressed in white shirts and navy shorts, they would stand still and stare at my daughter Lynda, a tall, skinny, fair-skinned 13-year-old with a blond pixie haircut. Where did this blond fairy come from, they seemed to wonder. Our bus later stopped at a park where a group of young boys were playing ball. Lynda was soon surrounded by all of them as she tried to teach them to finger whistle. What fun they all had!

We boarded the ship after it was provisioned in Kobe, and off we sailed to Hong Kong for a three-day visit. Again, we were overwhelmed by the Orient, its people, their customs, and traditions.

One experience in Hong Kong was set in motion the previous winter and was due to an upcoming Royal event. I knew that during our exciting year in England, as a Commonwealth exchange teacher, I would be invited to a Royal Tea at Buckingham Palace. I badly needed fancy clothes and accessories to attend this prestigious social event.

Fortunately, during that earlier winter, Lynda and I had enrolled in an art class in Vancouver where Lynda had befriended a young Chinese student named Gina, whose mother, Mrs. Chiu, lived in Hong Kong. Gina felt that her mother would be only too happy to help us with our shopping while in Hong Kong. Also, her mother dealt in pearls. I made arrangements with her that we would meet.

The morning the *Iberia* docked in Hong Kong, I phoned Gina's mother to confirm our plans. Mrs. Chiu was friendly and conveniently arranged for a taxi to deliver us to her home.

Before going to Mrs. Chiu's, Lynda and I joined a group of passengers on a morning tour to explore a local mountain. As we climbed up a steep path, the tour guide pointed out the strong wind blowing the bushes. He forecasted that a typhoon or tornado was coming our way. "Coming our way" gave no indication of time, and none of us knew much about typhoons, so we innocently proceeded with our agenda for the day.

Lynda and I joined Mrs. Chiu for lunch in a restaurant that she had selected. How different and how delicious were all the dishes Mrs. Chiu chose for us. We felt so humble and so grateful for her gracious hospitality. After lunch, she ushered us back to her office to discuss buying pearls. We were in awe when a fellow I will call "Mr. Pearl Man" opened his suitcase and uncovered a multitude of exquisite, dazzling round balls of various size, colour, and quality. I was truly dumbfounded, and I hesitated to make a choice. After

Mrs. Chiu was acquainted with our financial circumstances, she stipulated the best choice for our two sets of pearls, the correct length and size of pearl for each necklace and earring set. I was indeed indebted to her for the care she took to do this for us.

Then off we went to purchase new clothes for my Royal engagement. Lynda and I followed Mrs. Chiu through a bustling fabric shop where, after some time, we chose material for two beautiful garments. One was a lovely two-piece coat and dress ensemble and the other a two-piece white lace top and skirt suit. The dressmaker measured me from top to bottom for the necessary calculations for the garments that she would sew overnight. After the typhoon, my two beautiful perfectly-fitted outfits arrived at our cabin. What service! What workmanship! How grateful could we be?

We spent the day on shore experiencing the sights and sounds of Hong Kong street life—the food vendors, busy markets and other famous tourist attractions like Rat Alley. Arriving at our ship around 11 p.m., we were alarmed to learn that a typhoon indeed was heading straight for Hong Kong and would reach the city by midnight. To be safe, the *Iberia* must sail out from shore to avoid crashing against the dock. We were asked to make a choice: stay on board and sail out of the harbour or remain on shore. The purser explained that these storms had occurred many times before and that, each time, he had sailed out to sea and returned to shore safely. Upon consultation, Lynda and I decided to remain on board ship and sail out with the brave purser.

After departing the dock, I returned to our cabin and tried to read in my bed while Lynda went out on deck to "get some fresh air" and watch the approaching storm. We believed that the outer edge of the storm was still far out to sea. The typhoon, however, had strengthened to its peak and was arriving on our doorstep at 150 mph.

I was settling into bed, thinking that being out from the harbour as we were, the typhoon might not be much of a bother. Boy, was I wrong! I felt the ship lurch violently to one side and I landed on the floor. In an instant, the ship heeled to its lower side from the force of the wind. My first impulse was to get Lynda. I threw on a sweater, not even thinking that my adventure outside could be life-threatening. I had never experienced a typhoon, and the purser's reassurance that all would be well had made me braver than I might have been if I had known what to expect. I opened the door and immediately careened against the opposite wall. The sea shanty 'What Shall We Do With a Drunken Sailor,' came to mind as I swayed and staggered down the passageway. The thought of finding Lynda flooded my brain as the constant rocking motion made me more and more fearful. The ship's lurching felt like the inside of a jerky ride at the fair, only this ride was uncontrollable and unpleasant.

I stepped onto the deck and was met with a strong wind that pressed me back against the doorway. I only had time to notice the deck furniture lined up like soldiers facing the inky sea wall when a fierce wave smashed the deck, soaking me in salt water. I slipped and slid toward the railing and held on as best I could, but everything was wet and difficult to grip.

Thunderclouds were encircling overhead, but I could only sense them in the darkness. The deck was now awash with the power of the ocean: the waves kept coming at the ship from all directions. This was no fun ride at the fair.

I turned a corner with the help of a swift current of air and saw Lynda sitting on one of the teak lounge chairs. The wind captured my voice as I called out to her. I managed to grab hold of a metal structure jutting out from the side of the ship and tried again. I shouted as hard as I could, 'LYNDA'. This time she heard me and turned and waved to me. I motioned to her to come in, but my arm failed to move properly and looked more like I was raising my hand in class to ask a question. She waved again and looked back at the sea. I gingerly let go of the metal post, but seized it as hard as I could when a huge wave rose like a mountain over us and lunged for Lynda. I screamed as a mass of water sucked her to the railing. She and her chair slid to the brink of being overboard as the mountain and all its water receded back to sea. I stared in wonder as she hauled herself up, soaked from head to toe, and slid to my side. We grasped each other's hands and maneuvered our way around the deck chair 'soldiers', some of which had been knocked overboard while others lay lopsided and helpless in a crumpled mess.

We returned safely to our cabin and dried off. Lynda's stomach would have preferred to be on deck, but I made her stay in her bunk until morning. The next day, she ventured to the dining room to find all of the tables and chairs roped together. Only a few passengers were up and around. I was only able to consume some tea and crackers in the cabin.

When we had sailed away from the harbour to 'avoid' the storm, we left behind many bewildered, fellow passengers who had disembarked to enjoy a dinner tour and who had returned to find the ship gone. The shock was temporary: hotel staff provided them with accommodations in the hotel lobby and supplied toothbrushes, soap, and towels. Fortunately, damage in the harbour was minimal and no one was hurt. What an adventure! The purser was correct in this regard: the enormous ship endured the effects of the typhoon and sailed calmly to Hong Kong the next day.

Later in the voyage, we stopped in Singapore and then Bombay (now Mumbai). We were eating breakfast when a Mr. and Mrs. Hunter, who lived in Bombay, came to call for us. I happened to be bringing some parcels from Mr. Hunter's sister, Marie, in Vancouver and arranged to meet them. A crew member said "the hunters" were looking for us. We experienced a little cultural miscommunication, and I took it to be that *hunters* were looking for us, perhaps to shoot us! My imagination scurried past my common sense. A few laughs arose from the misunderstanding. The Hunters treated us to a sumptuous luncheon at their house, and we laughed over the scare since I knew they were quite innocent!

I believe that travellers, especially novice, naïve, and inexperienced ones must always be vigilant. Lynda and I, at that time, tried to be aware and to make each encounter tolerable and safe. I have tried to retain that advice in my head and heart and, to date, I have enjoyed many pleasant journeys by air and sea.

After departing from Bombay and a stop in Aden, our ship sailed up the Red Sea to Port Said, Egypt. Lynda and I disembarked to join a Cairo bus tour visiting the Pyramids and Sphinx. From the bus window, we were amused to see how our enormous ship seemed to glide through the sand as it was sailing up the Red Sea and then through the Suez Canal to Alexandria. The *Iberia* would be one of the last ships to go through the Suez Canal for some time due to the 1966 war in the Middle East.

On the last leg of the journey, we sailed the Mediterranean Sea to Barcelona, Spain. We went through the Straits of Gibraltar to Lisbon, Portugal, north along the west coast of France and across the English Channel into Southampton. We collected our luggage from the ship and said farewell to the *Iberia,* our home away from home for seven weeks.

In London we stayed at a bed and breakfast. Time went by quickly with sight-seeing and whatever else two naïve, novice travellers can experience in only four days in the great city of London.

At last, Lynda and I boarded the bus that would take us to Nuneaton, England, where I would be teaching second form students for the next ten months while their former teacher would teach my grade 2 class at Suncrest School in Burnaby. Lynda would pass two academic admission tests and would be studying at Nuneaton Grammar High School for girls.

My students and I got along just fine, but I could not quite understand their accents. I occasionally met their mothers and fared no better. One day a child from another class appeared at my classroom door asking, "May I have the book it, please, miss?" The little lad tried to communicate what he wanted three times, but still I could not understand what he needed, so I showed him in and said, "Please help yourself." He picked up a bucket and left. As time went on, the whole situation improved greatly, and we managed to communicate rather well.

The Royal Tea at Buckingham Palace Gardens was exciting and grand. Princess Alexandra, the youngest granddaughter of King George V and Queen Mary, was a gracious hostess as she greeted some 50 exchange teachers from the different Commonwealth countries. She made us feel welcome. What a great pleasure and honour to have been so lucky to attend such a lovely event. I looked nice in my new blue silk dress and matching coat, pearls, and white gloves, the wardrobe that was specially tailored for me in Hong Kong. Unfortunately, children were not invited to the Royal Tea, so Lynda could not attend the event.

During the course of the year, Lynda and I traveled extensively through Europe. We attended a wedding in Scotland, invited by the Canadian brother of the bride to take his place because he could not attend. For fall break, we went to Madrid, Spain and learned that people have a siesta at noon, dinner at 8 or 9 p.m., and then party into the wee hours. In Worchester we went shopping for china, and attended festivals and concerts. On most Sundays, we attended church services in Coventry.

During Christmas break in 1966, I was fortunate to join the Student's Union Club and travel to Russia. My roommate was from Australia, and she was excited to see snow for the first time in her life. The sights and sounds of Russia were intriguing and interesting. Language was not a problem for me being of Ukrainian descent, and I thought I was able to converse easily in Russian. One evening, however, my ability to communicate proved to be unsuccessful. A group of 14 students and I took the underground metro to a Philharmonic concert on the other side of Moscow, and had a thoroughly enjoyable evening. On the way back to our hotel, we stuck together for safety reasons, standing on the subway platform not quite knowing which train to board. Since I was the oldest and the only one knowledgeable, I thought, in the Russian language, I approached a comrade standing on the platform and, in Ukrainian, asked him whether we were on the right train track to get back to our hotel. He looked at me in dismay and exclaimed "*nyet, nyet, nyet*", looking at me over his shoulder as he hurried away. When I came back to my group to explain what had transpired, my Australian mate laughed and said: "You never know: perhaps he thought Mrs. Kotelko was inviting him back to her hotel!"

During the two-week Easter Spring school break, Lynda and I travelled on a bus tour of Israel visiting Tel Aviv, Haifa, the Sea of Galilee, Bethlehem and, of course, Jerusalem where we walked the

Stations of the Cross. We also had the opportunity to float in the Dead Sea.

When my teaching year in Nuneaton was over, we still had a period of time before sailing back to Vancouver. Lynda and I had planned a month-long bus tour of Europe, and in our busy itinerary not many countries would be spared. We were having a great time. At one town, I purchased enough material to make matching dresses for Lynda and me. After dinner in the hotel room, the two dresses were sketched and cut out with much care, stitched up by hand, and hemmed. No ironing was necessary. To complete the mother and daughter matching dresses we needed belts. I cut three long strips of fabric for each dress, and the next day, while we travelled from city to city, Lynda and I braided the two belts. That evening, there we were, mother and daughter in identical new dresses sashaying down the great staircase for dinner much to the delight and wonder of our travelling companions.

Our year away was almost over. For the final portion of our trip, Lynda and I boarded another great P&O passenger liner, the *Oriana* at Southampton, to sail across the Atlantic to Vancouver via the Panama Canal. In four weeks, we would be back to our normal lives, and I would be back in my own classroom. The international adventure and experiences would be forever treasured.

While Lynda and I were away in England, my older daughter Nadine attended Simon Fraser University in the education program. She had arranged for four university students to live in our house and help her with living expenses by paying room and board. Nadine had some challenges when she learned that one student was suicidal, one was a vegetarian, and another one was schizophrenic. What kind of meals could she provide these complicated roommates?

She soon sorted out the problems, dismissed her roommates, and returned to her pre-boarders' life, which entailed living on her own, while holding down two evening jobs, and excelling in her studies at SFU.

It was great to be back on home ground, back to a normal life, and the routine with family, friends, and neighbours. Thank the good Lord for guiding Lynda and me, and Nadine, on our endeavours and for blessing us with good health.

Flying around the world on 37 cents

I had caught the travel bug and on my next international expedition, called "Project Overseas", I was able to fly around the world at a cost to me of 37 cents.

In 1970, eight Canadian teachers and administrators were selected by the Canadian Teachers Federation and assigned to "Teach the Teachers" in Uganda, Africa for five weeks during the summer. Four educators were from B.C., one from Alberta, two from Ontario, and one from Québec. We assembled in Ottawa for a two-day orientation session on how to teach in Africa, and then spent two days in Rome attending university lectures in math and science. We landed at Entebbe International Airport in Kampala, Uganda and proceeded to the Tea House on the university campus where we would live comfortably for the next five weeks. One rule was strongly emphasized: we were not to venture outdoors after sundown because possible dangers lurked invisible in the dark of night.

We were scheduled to meet the rest of the staff at University Hall and were assigned a class of local teachers as our students. In a sense, I would call this a seminar. My job was to teach art with the help of another Canadian teacher from Toronto. Realizing how artistically creative Africans are we wondered how two Canadians could make a difference. Art materials were limited; therefore, we had to improvise. We created a mosaic using seeds of different colors and sizes. Our art display proved to be a great success.

An African safari to the Lake Victoria region involved camping outdoors. During the night, a herd of elephants roamed around us, stomping, sniffing, and snorting to their enjoyment and our amazement while we shivered in fear inside our tents. When we returned after an exhausting day to our hotel, we hurried into the pub to quench our thirst with beer, consumed in one gulp without stopping for a breath. We found the African heat unbearable even though it was actually their winter.

During an interesting discussion, a native African teacher said he hoped that our Quebec teacher would take at least four of his children back to Canada to be educated. He had 21 children at the time, and was not able to provide the necessities of life for all of them. Of course, the Canadian teacher was not able to help in such a personal family matter other than to recommend a family planning course, which, in this gentleman's case, was already too late.

A Roman Catholic priest from Toronto, who was part of our group, expressed a wish to return to Canada via the Orient. My art teaching partner Val and I decided to join him and fly from Kampala, Uganda to Bangkok, Thailand and then on to Vancouver. My travel agent adjusted and arranged my flight. All I needed to add to the cost of the original ticket provided by the Canadian Teachers Federation was 37 cents. What a great deal!

Yes indeed, I caught the travel bug early in life, and it is one happy germ I hope never to cure. That's one of the main reasons I love competing in track and field competitions around the world. Travelling, especially on the water, makes me feel alive and grateful for the sights, sounds, and sensations this wonderful world has to offer.

One recent memorable voyage coincided with the XVI World Masters Athletics Championships taking place in Riccioni, Italy in September 2007, when I was 88 years of age. While I was going abroad and on the way to Italy for the sports competition, I decided to try an intriguing way of water travel. I had heard about river cruising, and I was curious to experience this new and interesting way of travelling. The 18-day trip from Paris, France to Budapest, Hungary took us through four countries: France, Germany, Austria and Hungary. Our ship, *MS Avalon Tranquility*, sailed up and down five different waterways: the Moselle River, the Rhine River, the Maine River, Maine-Danube Canal, and finally the famous Danube River, sightseeing 13 different cities.

When I say up the river, that is, we sailed up the river as it flows downward from the mountains. At the numerous locks, the ship was raised to new levels and continued sailing up to the Maine-Danube canal. Then it was across the lock to where the Danube River flows downward, and the ship was lowered at the various locks until finally docking in Budapest. What a glorious 18-day trip, with the most appropriate name: the Jewels of Central Europe.

After the river cruise, I flew on to Riccioni, Italy where I competed in all of my regular events/disciplines. I brought home 8 gold medals and 1 silver medal, and wonderful memories of a remarkable expedition.

Today as I am writing about my river cruising adventure, news from Central Europe confirms that the 2013 spring floods are their worst floods of all time. Many river ships in Europe had to cancel trips, and were busing passengers and moving ships that were already full to alternate routes.

Since my cruise in 2007, river cruising has become a popular mode of travel. If you do decide to try it, you may want to keep in mind what savvy travellers suggest: Read the fine print in your booking paperwork. A river cruise is what you purchased, but a river cruise may not be what you get. Purchase travel insurance that allows you to cancel for any reason. And if you book your own air travel, leave enough time for any delays and glitches. People who thought they would be flying out of Prague were being bused to Munich.

These are some things to consider when you are planning your trip. The 2013 flood is not the first time Europe's rivers have flooded, and it won't be the last.

Your homework assignment:

How are you feeling about your life now? What gives you energy and lifts your spirits?

Did you know that many people who work out in the morning before work find their energy levels are higher throughout the day? Try it.

Make an inventory of all the things you love to do. I love to travel, to explore, and to meet new people. Do you know what truly brings you joy? If you have not figured that out at this stage in life, it's not too late. There is still time! Live in the moment. Be conscious of the journey and set your sights on what is best for you.

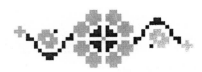

A little girl was talking to her teacher about whales.

The teacher said it was physically impossible for a whale to swallow a human because even though it was a very large mammal its throat was very small.

The little girl stated that Jonah fell into the ocean and was swallowed by a whale.

Irritated, the teacher reiterated that a whale could not swallow a human; it was physically impossible.

The little girl said, "When I get to heaven I will ask Jonah."

The teacher asked, "What if Jonah went to hell?"

The little girl replied, "Then you ask him."

Five

Sports & Athletics:
My New Passion

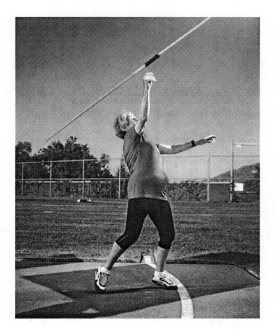

What precision! Patrik took the photo as I released
the javelin at just the right moment, aiming for that
tiny cloud in the sky. Patrik Giardino photo.

Lesson: Sport provides opportunities to learn about discipline, desire, determination, accomplishment, and success. The choice between team sports and individual sports branches into the diverse options in the sporting fields. Once you get out socializing and competing, you discover a new self-care practice that is healthy and fun. Competition is healthy. Set your sights on winning. The happiest and healthiest people are the ones who get out there and socialize.

"To dare is to lose one's footing momentarily. To not dare is to lose oneself."
— *Soren Kierkegaard*

Eleven siblings readily made two good teams for any game, be it softball, wolf & geese, anti-anti over, short stick/long stick, or a game we invented on the spot. Every game offered the chance for challenge and championship. Serious competition was at hand. To determine the equality and strength of the teams, we employed a strategy in making up the two sides, taking into consideration the age and sex of each player: fair is fair was our aim.

After supper, evening chores, and clean up, the Saskatchewan summer beckoned us for a competitive sport challenge before bedtime. The chirping birds in the nearby bulrushes were our cheerleaders and, after we tumbled into our beds, their enchanting choir eventually lulled us to sleep.

As I mentioned previously, after our two-mile walk to school each morning (warm up to our 8 a.m. brain work), we would enjoy a good game of softball or football if we could repair the lame equipment. Back in the 1930s and 1940s little, if any, organized sports were available. Not only did this lack prevent the introduction of team work and fitness for both boys and girls, the authorities discouraged females from taking part in rigorous sports. Why? Because they feared the girls would damage their reproductive organs.

After school, we formed our baseball team of five to seven boys and two girls. Mary Scherban and I would challenge the neighbouring school team six miles away. After our win, we walked home, jubilant, exhausted, and confident. What fun! Through team work, we learned and exhibited the challenge, determination, sportsmanship, and leadership required for sports.

Indeed, it was encouraging to become the champion softball team, from Riel Dana School, at our District Sports Days in Vonda.

The early benefits of team sports included the determination to succeed. This version of goal setting helped me when I determinedly completed my education so I could work as a teacher. While teaching for four years in Saskatchewan rural schools, I taught my students—farm children from ages 5-17—to become leaders, play fair, and be good sports. Later, during my teaching career in Burnaby, B.C., I saw how important athletics is for the health and development of all children. For my own health and well-being as a single parent, I pursued evening classes in yoga, tai chi, line dancing, and square dancing, while devoting time to enjoy my two daughters. Nadine would go on to teach with the Burnaby School Board for 20 years, and Lynda would became a paralegal.

I loved my teaching career; however, by law I was obliged to retire from teaching in 1984 at the age of 65. I wasn't sad or depressed, but it was unfortunate because I loved teaching, and I still had a lot of energy. The biggest change after retiring from the world of teaching came in 1989 when I moved from New Westminster to West Vancouver to live with Lynda, her husband Richard, and their two wonderful children, Matthew and Alesa. I was happy to live with them and to help with their growing family.

Never one to sit still, and with my family's encouragement, I became involved in the local West Vancouver Senior Centre. Immediately, I joined the Ramblers hiking club. Walking is a phenomenal form of exercise: you get the heart elevated while working some of the biggest muscles in your body. I attended an aqua fit class three times a week and continued to participate in yoga classes, painting classes, line dancing, and pottery. For my brain, I learned to play bridge. My life was full.

Bowling is a sport I enjoy immensely! When you think about it, a bowling alley is a little community centre where people enjoy friendship, fitness, and fun. From 1960–1984, every Thursday at 4 p.m., I played 10-pin bowling at Brentwood Lanes with the Burnaby Teachers Bowling Club. We occupied all 48 lanes. I was punctual and dedicated to the sport and developed great skill and technique to maintain a substantial average of 150+.

Our team record states: "Olga demonstrated good sportsmanship and leadership. She enjoyed strong health habits of balance, poise and camaraderie. Olga was a joyful athlete in the bowling club and was admired for her spirit and a role model."

From 1988–2002, I bowled 10-pin weekly in three leagues with the Happy 55 Gang at Brunswick Lions Gate Bowling Lanes in West Vancouver. I continued my membership with the Happy 55 Gang at Rev's Bowling Centres in Burnaby, B.C., (formerly Brentwood Lanes) when the West Vancouver bowling lanes closed. I maintained an average of 146 at the age of 86, and at the age of 93 my average was 127. Pretty good.

I soon decided to pursue the game of slo-pitch softball. I was thankful that the North Shore Saltchuckers Slo-Pitch Team signed me up. Slo-pitch is a form of softball played with eight men and two women on each side, and in which each pitch must travel in an arc 3-10 feet high. Base stealing is not permitted.

Initially, I detested the sport because I was unable to connect my bat with the ball. I persevered and persisted, however, and eventually I came to love the game with a passion. I enjoyed the competition and the camaraderie while competing against teams in and around Vancouver. The joy of winning games on a sports team filled a void in my athletic life.

I played a number of positions: catcher, 1st, 2nd, and 3rd base, shortstop, and right field. I liked playing 2nd base the best. People began to notice me when I played and, as I mentioned previously, I showed up on the sport's radar when I made a double play that put out runners at 1st base and home plate.

I loved slo-pitch softball, especially because I played well in every position, but age became a factor in my decision to leave the game. One day, during a particularly intense game, I was backing up to catch a fly ball. Suddenly, a male centre fielder who was twice my size tackled me; he thought the ball was his to catch. Ouch, that hurt! I soon realized it was time to leave the game to younger blood. I had played until 1996 at the age of 77 and loved it. A short time after retiring from softball, I turned my attention to track and field, and chose running and throwing events not unlike those skills necessary in softball.

I branched off to track and field on the advice of my mentors, Bob Robinson, and fellow slo-pitch player, Al Jarvis. These two men were physical education teachers and coaches at North Shore schools. Bob had coached the legendary athlete Harry Jerome in the 1960s. These two men believed in me. They believed I could do it; therefore, I worked for it.

Every Tuesday and Thursday we went to the high school track and worked on track and field events. I had a few things to learn. For instance, when I approached local high schools for some throwing equipment I didn't realize, until I was asked what sizes I wanted, that the shot put, discus and javelin came in specific dimensions. I took home what was available. At first, throwing the javelin, shot put, and discus was a challenge; I had never seen nor held these intriguing instruments. Off to the library I went to learn more about these implements. I also carefully watched other people demonstrate their skills at various track and field championships. With their guidance, I started to practice throwing the javelin, shot put, and discus with a vengeance.

The coaching I received, from Al, Bob, and later Barb Vida, trained me to achieve my objectives. Their coaching, training, and instructing gave me self-awareness of track and field events, and they offered methods of improvement that I could not have worked on without their help. I benefitted from their critique of my form, their keen eyes for detail, and their encouragement when I was feeling less than 100%.

When I turned my attention to athletics, I channeled the same concentration that I put into teaching. I pursued and persisted and became proficient in my new athletic career, a career that I treasure with all of my heart. I joined the Canadian Masters Athletic Association. Membership in the CMA is open to anyone who is interested in masters and sub-masters fitness. "Masters" are defined as women and men 35 and over. Masters championships' competition is limited to those ages, in 5-year age sets, up to the age of the oldest competitor. The North Shore Nor-Westers Track and

Field Club helped me with the 100 m sprint, shot put, javelin, and discus throw. Coach and trainer Barb Vida helped me to develop the specific technique and skill in those events. I also perfected the hammer and weight throws, weight pentathlon, 200m, 400m, high jump, long jump, and triple jump.

Barb diligently continued to guide, encourage, and instruct with a firm hand for a couple of years. We started warm-ups with ABC drills of strength training and a form of injury prevention as well. Drills train muscles to "fire faster" and help the legs work more efficiently. Barb introduced me to the exercise machines at the gym to develop general and core strength for jumps, sprints, and throws. She was a wonderful coach. Soon I felt capable to train and compete on my own. In 1997, I competed against five other senior competitors in the B.C. Senior Games in the 75-79 years of age category. There was no other way to go but up!

"The spirit of a true athlete does not simply show in competition but in practice as well," said Barb. Barb's coaching and encouragement enabled me to become extremely dedicated in the gym through a program of consistent exercise, which included general and functional weight training and cardio training, in addition to my track and field technical training.

Senior athletes throwing a javelin, doing the long jump, or running do not have access to their own tracks; consequently, Barb and I would drive around for miles to find an empty school track. Prior to any actual training, my warm-up consisted of me using my spade to dig a pit for the long and triple jumps. For high jump, I needed separate equipment that was seldom available, so high jump came later in my program.

I am neither a coach nor a trainer, but I can share with you my personal training regime. I can show and advise you how and where to start the journey in track and field.

Two months prior to a competition I start training for my 9 to 12 different disciplines. Only in fair weather (not when it's raining), I spend 2 to 3 hours training outdoors by myself, mainly at West Van Senior Secondary School (WVSS) and other neighbourhood schools.

> Warm up—alternate walking slow laps, fast laps on the track;
>
> Warm up—running slow laps, fast laps on the track;
>
> Sprint 50m-75m—increase distance with rest;
>
> Combine 1-2 throws events with 1-2 jump events;
>
> Cool down by again walking or jogging.

Monday, Wednesday, and Friday, I alternate my OK exercises and aquafit three times a week, with training at WVSS on Tuesday, Thursday, and Saturday. On rainy days, I train in the gym. On Sundays, I go to church to give thanks for all my blessings.

My first international masters competition was at the age of 78 in Tucson, Arizona. From May 21-28, 1997, I joined 10,000 athletes taking part in the National Senior Olympic Sports Classic. I was honoured to be chosen to carry the Canadian flag into the enormous Tucson University Stadium and lead the Canadian contingent of 72 athletes. When I competed in Tucson, I was in the 75-79 age group.

The javelin required for the competition weighed only 400 grams, 200 grams lighter and slightly shorter than the one I had practiced with at home. My 5th throw measured 57 feet. The judge announced that the other competitors had to beat that number. My 6th throw was an amazing 19.94 m (65'5"), which was 15 feet farther than the second place finisher. It felt as if an angel had picked up my javelin and carried it that far. With that throw, I broke the World and American records and established a new Canadian record.

The other competitors swarmed around to congratulate me. "What do you eat? How much do you train? Do you have a coach? How much do you sleep?" They plied me with question after question. The official, a former world javelin athlete, inquired about where I was from, saying that he liked my style of performance. He told me that I had great potential.

The walk to the podium to receive my first gold medal in a track and field competition was an exhilarating experience. Sheer ecstasy! I have gone on to win more than 600 gold medals in my athletic career, but I will always remember that day in Tuscon. I had won my first international gold medal; I was hooked. I realized that I loved track and field; I loved competing; I especially loved the feeling of camaraderie among the athletes.

Earlier in the day, while strolling around the track, a man walked by me and said, "Well, that's a winner if I ever saw one!" I looked down on my chest, and I saw that my competition number was 777. What a lovely coincidence: I'm the seventh of eleven children. Seven must be my lucky number. I guess I did something fantastic that day.

The success of my new athletic career encouraged me to challenge myself more, so I began competing in local, national, and international championships. In 1999, at the age of 80 years, I competed in 9 local, national, and international championships. The World Masters Athletics Championships in Gateshead England was my first World Track and Field Meet abroad. With trepidation, I anticipated competing against more experienced, seasoned, and former Olympic athletes. Luckily, I blended in with the crowd of almost 6,000 athletes from 74 countries, of which 134 participants were from Canada. The whole experience was truly one of a kind. The sounds of all the different languages from various countries made the experience all the more exciting.

The first day I competed in the hammer throw and 100m sprint in the woman's 80-84 age group. I earned a gold medal in each event. The next day was the shot put competition where I received a third gold medal. The excitement in me was building, overcoming my initial fear as I realized that I could throw farther and run faster than the big, muscular, more experienced German and Russian athletes. The momentum continued throughout the competition.

I came home with a total of 8 gold and 2 silver medals. I also set two World Records for the high jump (92cm) and weight pentathlon (3721 points).

The experience was incredible and not one to be forgotten. Many of the athletes asked where I had been for the past years and why I had not been competing with them. I told them I wasn't aware that this kind of competition even existed. The encouragement and camaraderie were a tremendous boost to my self-esteem. After a number of years being a retired teacher, I had now discovered an exciting path that led to a new and untapped version of myself at the age of 78. I was a champion athlete, a competitor that could win medals. I happily identified with this new image of myself, an identity that I planned to nurture for the rest of my life.

To date, at the age of 95, I have amassed 9 bronze medals, 21 silver medals, and over 700 gold medals. I don't hoard them in boxes behind the chesterfield; I give them away as gifts for anniversaries, birthdays, rewards for good deeds, and at our church bazaars. One day, 63 people participated in a church sports' event; at another event, 74 international delegates attended a Vancouver convention and each of them received a gold medal.

My journey as a serious athlete began 13 years after retiring from my teaching career. I chose to become a young-at-heart athlete rather than an old woman. Today I have more energy, more strength, more stamina, and more spirit than ever before, and I feel great!

I do this to stay flexible and to maintain good health in body, mind and spirit.

Being a track and field athlete provides the strength and endurance to keep my body healthy. I continue to train outdoors, on my own, at a local high school track and field facility, when it is not raining. I have learned to prepare properly for each of the track and field events I enter and, when executed in the right way, those events can result in success every time. Stan Jensen, a trainer, maintained that "if you under-train, you might not finish; if you over-train, you might not start". I feel I am quite proficient in the skills I have acquired for competitions. I need only to maintain my endurance. Both aerobic and endurance training provide the greatest benefits for reducing blood pressure.

Once you get serious about competing, training is no longer a chore. It's what makes you happy. It becomes a near obsessive way of life. You want to get into the shot put ring knowing you did more and are better prepared than the other athletes. And what draws people into the ring is a high like no other. You step in, and you can't even hear the crowd cheering. You're thinking about the record of the best throw so far. It's the ultimate rush; you're putting everything you have at risk to prove you've trained harder and you want it more. Beecher Riesin, trainer from the Champion Martial Arts Academy in North Vancouver, describes it well: "You know if you lose you can get eliminated. If you win, you've conquered success."

I measure and account for all the moments when I am most happy as a competitive athlete. I keep exact records of all my track and field competitions. I place great importance on the measurement of my progress. Why? Because I need to know what I am able to achieve. If I can't measure it, I can't manage it.

If you look after the little things, sometimes the big things take care of themselves. Track and field is my passion, and currently I hold 26 world records. My track and field events consist of the following:

> Sprints—100m, 200m, 400m, 800m;
>
> Jumps—high jump, long jump, triple jump;
>
> Throws—shot put, discus, javelin, hammer, weight;
>
> Pentathlon—hurdles, long jump, shot put, high jump and 800m;
>
> Throws Pentathlon—weight, hammer, shot put, discus, javelin;
>
> Relays—4 x 100m, 4 x 200m, 4 x 400m.

These are the events in which I compete, but there are many other different and various sports events a person could choose from. Track and field competitions also include hurdles, pole vault, distance walking, and running.

Games' championships are composed of some 26 or more different sports, beginning with archery. Ball sports include baseball, basketball, bowling, golf, racquetball, softball, tennis, table tennis, and volleyball. Other sports are badminton, cycling, horseshoes, race walking, road racing, shuffleboard, swimming, and triathlon. If you need a challenge to keep fit, make your choice, have fun, and go for it. Use it or lose it! If you need help, email me. Hurdles, pole vault, distance walking, and running are great events.

There had not been any jumps records for women in the 90–94 age group as no one in that age category had ever tried competing in these events. At age 90, I established World Records in high jump (0.82 meters), long jump (1.77 meters) and triple jump (4.25 meters). I challenge other women to strive to beat these records because I believe all records are made to be broken. I'm not easily impressed with my own fame, but people see my stats and stats don't lie. Thank you for helping me build my spirit. I hope to jump when I turn 95 and 100. God willing.

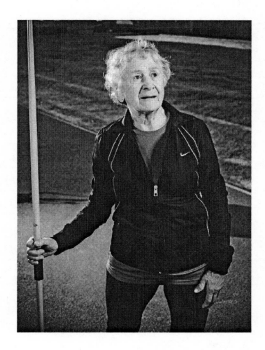

Be ready for your turn. Patrik Giardino photo.

It was in March 2010 that I received an invitation for study and research from Dr. Tanja Taivassalo, researcher at McGill University Kinesiology Department. Dr. Taivassalo had attended the World Outdoor Masters 2009 Track and Field Championship in Lahti, Finland and watched me compete at 90 years of age. She and her team were anxious to test my physical abilities in the Montreal lab. I have included the Montreal episode in the Community chapter.

The writer, Bruce Grierson, arranged a trip for me to meet with Dr. Art Kramer and his staff at Beckman Institute, University of Illinois in Chicago. The researchers peeked into my brain while a battery of tests—23andMe Genetic Health Overview was performed. This commentary is highlighted also in the Community chapter. *What Makes Olga Run* by Bruce Grierson will be published in January 2014.

My World Track and Field Records as of August 2013, compiled by Harold Morioka, B.C. Representative to the Canadian Masters Athletics Association.

Sport	Categ.	Record	Age	Date	Location
Outdoor Records					
200 m	W90	56.46	90	03.08.09	Lahti, Finland
400 m	W90	2:50.28	90	17.09.09	Richmond, BC
High Jump	W85	0.94m	85	28.08.04	Dorado, PUR
	W90	0.82m	90	01.08.09	Lahti, Finland
Long Jump	W90	1.77m	90	07.08.09	Lahti, Finland
Triple Jump	W90	4.25m	90	18.09.09	Richmond, BC
Discus Throw	W90	14.80m	90	06.08.09	Lahti, Finland
Shot Put	W90	5.43m	91	17.09.10	Courtenay, B.C.
Hammer Throw	W90	16.71m	92	08.07.11	Sacramento, CA
Javelin Throw	W85	18.56m	85	26.06.04	Eugene, OR

	W90	13.54m	90	03.08.09	Lahti, Finland
Weight Throw	W90	7.90m	90	17.09.10	Courtenay, BC
Throws Pentathlon	W85	4211 pts	85	18.07.04	Calgary, AB
	W90	4287 pts	90	06.08.09	Lahti, Finland
4 x 100 Metres	W80+	1:49:15	CAN	13.09.08	Prince George, BC
Indoor Records					
60 Metres	W90	15.14	91	02.03.10	Kamloops, BC
200 Metres	W90	60.72	91	03.03.10	Kamloops, BC
400 Metres	W90	3:31.50	93	08.04.12	Jyvaskyla, Finland
800 Metres	W90	8:49.15	93	03.04.12	Jyvaskyla, Finland
High Jump	W85	0.89m	85	14.03.04	Sindelfingen
	W90	0.76m	93	07.04.12	Jyvaskyla, Finland
Long Jump	W85	1.91m	85	13.03.04	Sindelfingen
	W90	1.70m	92	20.03.11	Kamloops, BC
Triple Jump	W85	4.06m	88	15.02.08	Kamloops, BC
	W90	4.14m	91	05.03.10	Kamloops, BC
Shot Put	W90	5.74m	92	19.03.11	Kamloops, BC
Weight Throw	W90	7.51m	92	20.03.11	Kamloops, BC
Pentathlon	W90	2326 pts	93	03.04.12	Jyvaskyla, Finland
4 x 200 Metres	w80+	4:15.33	CAN	06.03.10	Kamloops, BC
Total *World Records*	26				

As I say, records are made to be broken. If I could jump at 89, why not jump at 90? I am so *grateful* to be able to do all of this at my age. It's still good for my body. Once you get serious about competing, you want to keep going. Go for the gold! For those of you who love numbers and stats, I have included all my athletic achievements from 2004 and 2009. You will find them at the end of the book.

Championships give me the opportunity to travel and compete. I have competed throughout Canada as well as in Argentina, Australia (4 times), Barbados, England, Finland (2 times), Germany, Italy (2 times), Mexico, Puerto Rico, Spain, and the United States (many times).

In October, I competed at the 2013 World Masters Athletics Championships in Porto Alegre, Brazil. I had earlier strained my right shoulder rotator cuff ligament while writing this book in longhand, and injured it further during the summer when I competed in three championships; consequently, I had to throw with my left hand. I was originally registered in 11 events, but had to scratch the Hammer Throw, not because of my injury, but because I couldn't get from one venue to the next within the 15 minute time requirement: a taxi took 40 minutes. Throws Pentathlon also had to be scratched because I had a sore throat, brought on by the cold, damp weather. As a result, I was only able to compete in 9 events for which I won 9 gold medals.

I also hope to compete in 2014 in Hungary, and in 2015 in Lyon, France. I love to compete, travel, and make new friends. Let me tell you about the time I received a phone call from a prince!

During the 2009 World Masters Games in Australia there was much jubilation for Ruth Frith who had turned 100. I wanted so much to see Ruth compete in track and field throws at her age. It was exciting that we would be meeting and celebrating her athletic performance, one that was super for her. Sunday, October 11, 2009 would be my last championship meet for the year 2009, the year I turned 90. I was the new kid on the block that year, being the youngest athlete in my age category W90-94. My performance was great; every sprint, jump, and throw produced a world record and earned a gold medal. As I had no competitors, it was my turn to break previous records as well.

HRH Prince of Malaysia presented me with one of my gold medals. Ordinarily, I don't hoard my medals in boxes and drawers, and I give them away as signs of appreciation. The prince was overwhelmed when I presented him with one of my newly acquired gold medals. We chatted for a while and had our picture taken. I mentioned that in February 2010, Vancouver would be hosting the Winter Olympics. He said he knew this and would be attending the games.

During the 2010 Olympics, I was involved with the Olympic Torch Relay organizers. I was assigned to carry the Olympic torch on February 12 at 7:45 p.m. in West Vancouver. The excitement was overwhelming. Lo and behold, it got better when I received a phone call from the assistant to the Prince of Malaysia who said the prince and his family were in Whistler, and he would like to speak with me. I was overjoyed with anticipation. I was kept in suspense for three long days, and I didn't leave the house even for aquafit class or to make pyrogies because "My Prince" would be calling.

Finally, on Sunday afternoon, the assistant called and said, "The prince would like to speak with you." I just about dropped the phone. A very pleasant voice said how happy he and his family were to be in Vancouver, especially in Whistler. What a great city and what hospitality, he said. He was having a wonderful time. I was practically speechless with excitement, and I thanked him for remembering that I lived in Vancouver. My prince had phoned me.

As much as I may like to speak with royalty, I am uncomfortable in the public eye. I just want to be a friend and quietly do my own thing. I have always been humble. In 2009 I was honoured to be inducted into the Canadian Master Athletes Hall of Fame. I try to relay my message to as many children and seniors as I can. If I can inspire some, there might just be that one in a crowd somewhere who will one day be in their own respective Hall of Fame.

What a treat to be selected for the Canadian Masters Athletics Hall of Fame, especially when I would be among the legends of track and field. My induction was such a huge honour and caught me a bit by surprise. I definitely didn't think about it when I was competing. With every competition, I always promise myself that I will win a medal. I don't say what colour.

When the time comes, that promise I made gives me more determination to go harder than the other athletes. When my body wants to stop because it hurts so much, I think of my promise. I work as hard as I possibly can. Throughout the competitions, because of my promise to work hard enough to win a medal, the bronze medal feels as good as the gold.

When I was inducted into the Hall of Fame, I heard the audience cheer. I had to pinch myself that I was a member of such an elite group of track and field athletes. What a special moment to realize I belonged with them. All the hard work, the family support, the dedication to improvement, and the ability to stay healthy contributed to my success. All that effort was important, but two things assisted me in attaining my athletic goals: my desire to stick to the training, and my love for the sport. I couldn't be prouder!

Even with this "Master Athlete of the Year" title, it's already behind me. That was in March 2010, being ranked by Sports B.C. Now I am thinking ahead, and I can't wait to turn 95 and enter the W95 category. Whatever I did, how high I jumped, world records, gold medals, all that is behind me. The biggest thing for me is to surpass the existing records and move on. Be positive: that is the best attitude.

Older adults, over 50, 60, and 70 years of age, are becoming serious athletes competing in local, national and international championships. These senior athletes are experiencing a level of fitness that can fight debilitating aging. This is the secret to staying young and healthy: our bodies were meant to move. When you feel fit, you are flexible, which is a natural feeling. Your body is balanced and co-coordinated with strong healthy bones and muscles. An active person can remain healthy and in the last years of life avoid a long bout of ill health. This is what we all should experience. I am referring mainly to athletes, because this is a world I know.

One of my fellow competitors, Earl Fee, a much sought after motivational speaker who has written a book entitled *How to be a Champion from 9 to 90* has this to say about longevity: "Who wouldn't be interested in living longer and at the same time enjoying higher quality living? Aging is affected by your genes, but your real biological age depends largely on your everyday habits of eating, sleeping, drinking, physical and mental exercising, stress level, smoking, etc. Slowing down is due more to rusting out than aging. Get rid of that 'I am slow because I'm old' thinking."

Here is one example of what determination and perseverance is all about in sport competition. Fellow competitor Soumé, W84, is 9 years younger than I. She and I ran a 200m sprint at USATP Championships in Lisle, Illinois in August 2012. Not being totally aware at the time of our age difference, I stayed with Soumé until about 25 metres to the finish line. I thought to myself why not add a little pressure, and I almost beat her. I might have passed her if I had added that little effort sooner. This was a good lesson.

There is always next time. It's good to have a challenge and to feel competitive.

I believe the reason I ran the 200m sprint with such ease was because I had 40 minutes before the race to lie on the grass and elevate my legs at a 45° angle against the fence. I could feel the energy returning to my legs when I most needed it. At the finish line, I was able to walk and talk with ease.

If sagging skin, faulty organs, arthritis, failing hearts and minds can develop from losing the battle against gravity, I feel I am winning that battle every time I push myself to run faster, jump higher, throw farther.

I am happy to be a mentor to women athletes who are following in my footsteps and embarking on a career of master competition in track and field events. Track and field is not ice skating. It's not necessary to smile and make a wonderful impression on the judges. Forget about looking cool. This is about survival in running, jumping, and throwing.

I love my new sports career. I love competing. I love travelling around the world. I love making new friends. I have no reason to stop. I have no plans to stop! I am enjoying my health and lifestyle, and I thank God that He keeps me healthy and gives me the opportunities to use my talent. It's kind of nice to win and to be recognized. I believe in an old Chinese saying, "It's not how old you are; it's how you get old." What a great life I have discovered, and I wish the same for you!

You are the champion. Keep everything simple. Just do what you do and trust how you do it. It's amazing how many elements determine a champion. The weight on your shoulders to carry your country is not a burden. All the caring and support will lift you and not weigh you down.

Go for it champ! You can do it! Trust yourself!

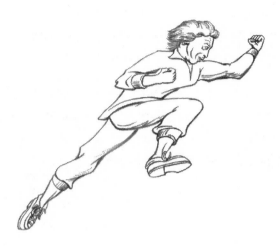

Gravity. We can't see it or touch it, but it guides our destiny. I want to defy gravity. Sketch by David Kind.

Your homework assignment:

Today, give your complete attention to physical activity. Observe how challenging it is to use your physical body in new and different ways. Persist and persevere when you encounter any difficulties.

Discover the fine balance between effort and exhaustion. Be competitive but don't gamble with your well-being. Wear good workout shoes that provide comfort and support.

Have the courage to discover what you need to do in order to stay healthy. Exercise is not a luxury; it is the key to healthy aging. Choose a physical activity that you enjoy, and if you need additional information, ask for help. Sports and age have no boundaries.

Get moving. Remember to stretch before working out. Stretching will improve the range of motion in your muscles and joints. If you're just beginning an exercise program, get a few weeks of strength training under your belt. Your aerobic or cardiovascular workouts will be much more enjoyable.

Don't set up barriers. Say to yourself: "If Olga can do it, I can do it!" I believe if there is a will, there is a way, and determination and discipline are the two key elements in achieving your goals. And remember, there is a first time for everything.

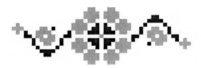

Our dishwasher has been broken for some time, so my husband, who is waiting for a knee replacement, does the dishes. I came home from work one evening very tired, and as we were cleaning up after dinner, I announced that one of these days I was going to get that dishwasher fixed. Our 7-year-old grandson Chris quick-wittedly piped in, "All it needs, Grandma, is a new knee".

Six
Why Community Matters

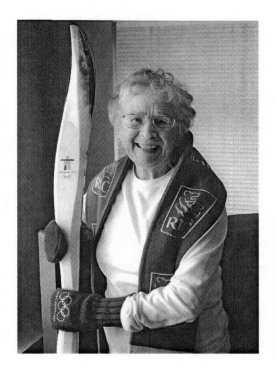

Carrying the torch in the 2010 Vancouver Olympic
Torch Relay. Noris Burdeniuk photo.

Lesson: The happiest, healthiest people in the world are the ones who socialize and stay close to the people they love and who feel loved and needed in return. Having friends will boost your well-being and provide you with the support you need during the most dire and difficult situations. Remember: even when things look very dark in your life, you can find the energy and inspiration to hang in there and get your life back together. Being a member of a vibrant community helps build and add to a happy, healthy lifestyle.

"Happiness is not the absence of problems; it's the ability to deal with them."

– Steve Maraboli

Without a doubt one of the highlights in my life was to be chosen as a torch bearer in the Vancouver 2010 Olympic Torch Relay. It was that once-in-a-lifetime experience, and it was wonderful to run my stage of the relay in my own neighbourhood of West Vancouver. On February 10 at 7:45 p.m., I ran along Marine Drive between 15th and 17th streets.

Three Canadian cities have played a role in my life: I was born and raised in Smuts, Saskatchewan; I raised my children and developed my teaching career in New Westminster; and now I am enjoying my retirement in West Vancouver.

My home town of Smuts was named by an executive of the Canadian National Railway after a British army officer when a railroad track was built from Melfort to Saskatoon. Although I called it home for almost 25 years and it was where I started my teaching career in a little one-room schoolhouse, I left town soon after I married only to return again as a visitor with my children for summer holidays. Like a number of other prairie towns, Smuts died out after train service was removed. The two grain elevators were closed, and the schools soon followed. This is the sad history of many towns and villages across Canada. Once the economic lifeblood of the community is removed, followed by the loss of townspeople, they quickly become ghost towns.

A number of years ago, someone reported the sighting of actual ghosts in Smuts. This report brought thrill seekers who caused a great deal of damage and vandalism to the old grocery store, the hotel, and to the church. Luckily, the teenage vandals were caught and punished. If there was an apparition sighted, it was most likely one of my cousins who lives in the neighborhood and who took on the responsibility of caring for the church. St. John the Baptist, a beautiful church considered a heritage site, can be seen like a beacon from miles around.

In the first chapter of my book, I recounted some early family memories. A family is the smallest unit of an organized community, and the need for solidarity and respect for each member means a willingness to cooperate. A family is a mini-community that is magically bonded together by ties of affection, loyalty, and mutual respect.

Of my 10 siblings, I am the only one still alive today. I think of my brothers and sisters fondly and consider myself fortunate to have loved each and every one of them. As the middle child in a large family, I occupied an excellent position to know and appreciate their different qualities and personalities.

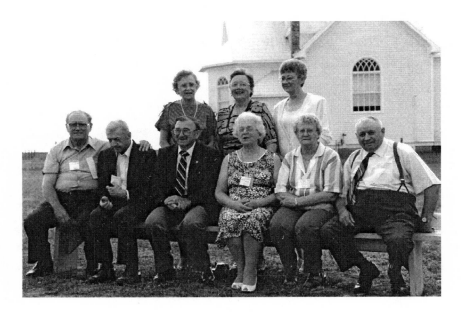

This photo was taken at the 1986 Shawaga Family Reunion.
Front row l to r: Mike, Steve, Matt, Jean Burdeniuk, Anne
Korpan, John. Standing l to r: Olga Kotelko, Phyllis Gutiw,
Kay Chomyn. Missing are dad and mom, of course, and eldest
sister Mary Parchewsky and youngest brother Alex.

After my eldest brother Mike retired from farming, he built and
operated a general store. He was an excellent manager. He became
a successful entrepreneur in Saskatoon, buying older homes, refur-
bishing them, and reselling them. He lived to be 90 years and
4 months.

I always looked up to my eldest sister, Mary, who was a gracious
lady. Everything that she did was a masterpiece, and cooking was
her specialty. I thoroughly enjoyed working with her in her home
and learning from her all that I now know about food preparation, sewing, knitting, and crocheting. Mary was also a successful
entrepreneur. She demonstrated leadership, was a great mentor, and

always had time to give advice and assistance. My interest in reflexology came from Mary. I miss her dearly.

Anne was great fun, and we shared a lot of laughs together. We always enjoyed shopping for bargains at garage sales and second-hand stores. She had a good eye for Canadian furniture and antiques of all sorts. Anne organized and hosted many great parties and was always a helpful friend.

Sister Jean was the great family seamstress. She loved to crochet and was good at creating new and different dress patterns for our mother and sisters. Jean liked to sew similar dresses for her and me. Once we attended a country barn dance dressed alike. I still remember the magenta velvet dress embroidered with beads that she sewed for me so that I would be pretty for my first day at school. She was a real treasure.

As I mentioned previously, our father had acquired a lot of land. Brother John was the farmer in the family. John and my other brother, Matt, would walk seven miles to a dance, enjoy the festivities all night long and then walk back home. After changing from their best clothes, they went to feed the horses and then got ready to spend the rest of the day out on the fields.

I recall one Christmas when I returned home from Saskatoon for the holidays. John and his friends came to meet me at the Smuts train station with a big sleigh pulled by two horses. As he drove home, he intentionally made a sharp turn very quickly, tipping over the sleigh and me under it. What fun! Luckily nobody was hurt, and I will always remember that sleigh ride and brother John, the prankster.

My brother Matt loved sugar. It was his elixir. He would wait around after supper until everybody had settled down to read, do homework, work on puzzles, or play cards, and he would discreetly open the cupboard and help himself to a spoonful of sugar. I caught him once, and he made me promise not to tell on him. I can do so now, Matt. He worked hard on the land and was a great helper to our parents. He was a kind soul, liked by everybody, and fun to have around. Matt was also a hell of a good baseball player. I believe it was because of Matt that our baseball team was the champion in the school district.

Brother Steve was the comedian, the entertainer in the family, and he loved horses. During the family reunion, he recalled how sad it was during the Depression to see the horses grow so thin. Steve loved to get out of work whenever and wherever. He wanted to play, which was often. One evening, he proceeded to put on a bicycle exhibition. He made the bike move forward as he stood on the seat with his hands on the handlebars. That was a great show for an 8-year-old. He could also hit homeruns in baseball.

Phyllis, the actress, had the talent to write, choreograph, and act out a skit or play that would include most of the 30-40 children in our rural schoolhouse. She provided the Friday afternoon entertainment that ended our school week. Phyllis was the jack-of-all-trades, a hostess, teacher, and provider. She was also handy around the house: always able to fix and repair things. Later in life, Phyllis became an hotelier: family and friends from afar knew where they could stay in Saskatoon when they came to visit.

Sister Kay was kind and polite, gentle and sweet. She was a cheerful companion who had a lot of friends. *Princess* Kay was the best name for her. Kay liked to coordinate what we would be wearing, from eyeglasses and even to the colour of our socks. She loved to entertain and to socialize. Very often I think how much fun we had. She died far too young.

The youngest of the Shawaga munchkins was Alex. One morning, Alex complained about his porridge because he didn't want to go to school that day. He wanted to eat rice. Mother knew the reason behind his act. She tricked him by saying she would serve him some other kind of breakfast. He decided better of his decision, ate the porridge, and hurried off to catch up with the rest of us. Alex was a happy and cheerful fellow. He was an exceptional athlete, bringing home more ribbons than the rest of us combined.

We all enjoyed sports from an early age. We played baseball in the summer, and wore out our sleds and skates in the winter. We were always moving. And, of course, there were all those daily farm chores like milking 15 cows by hand, separating 5-7 large pails of milk, washing clothes by hand on the scrub board, and then walking the two miles to school. My family benefitted from a healthy lifestyle and our motto was *"Work hard / Play hard"*.

Believe it or not, I really enjoyed ironing, especially men's white dress shirts. You may think: "What a thing to enjoy!" But I became good at it, much to the benefit of my father and five brothers. With so many men in the family, there was a lot of ironing. Remember, this was before electricity. I used a flat iron heated on a wood burning stove.

I don't remember whose idea it was, but we decided it was time for a family reunion. In July, 1986, the Shawaga clan reunited to celebrate the 85th anniversary of our family's arrival in Canada. It was a grand event and attracted 200 immediate family members from across North America. The three-day weekend included a family supper, dance, talent show, as well as organized games, photo sessions, and a breakfast with bread baked in a newly built outdoor clay oven.

There was a lot of laughter mingled with a few tears as I reunited with my brothers and sisters. Mom and dad were sorely missed. The 1986 family reunion was an opportunity for us to relive those happy early years, the "good old days". We recaptured the true flavour of early family life on the farm. We spent days building a *peech*, the outdoor oven, pioneer style, in a field adjacent to the church. The smell of homemade bread wafting from an outdoor oven is medicine for the soul. The *peech* would be our legacy.

A frame was molded into a tunnel shape. Stomping feet were used to knead the clay, straw, and water into mud. The mud was then used to cover the tunnel inside and out, leaving one end open as the oven door. I was elected to work on the inside, and I remember the mud collapsed on me a couple of times. But perseverance by all got the job done. Next came the drying process that consisted of building low fires for a few days until the *peech* was dry.

To bake in the oven, we built a large fire and then we removed the hot, white coals. The baker checked the oven periodically until the temperature was just right for baking. On reunion day, the *peech* was put to the test and passed beautifully. We enjoyed freshly baked, homemade bread as well as beet-leaf *holubtsy*, called *beetnicks*.

Our large, happy, family event was documented by second and third generation family members, Anne Gutiw, Carol Issel and Bernice Shawaga.

> *Family ties and connections were always of great importance to all Shawaga family members. In July 1986, over 200 family members from all across North America congregated at the small town of Smuts, which was the hub of family activity 100 years ago, and on that weekend.*

This town is about one mile from the original Shawaga homestead. Three generations were represented: the children of Anna and Wasyl Shawaga, their grandchildren and great grandchildren. We assembled to appreciate our family heritage; our strengths and successes were a legacy from our original immigrant homesteaders.

Three days over the weekend included a family supper, dance, talent show and organized games, photo sessions and a breakfast with bread baked in a newly built outdoor clay oven. All family members enjoyed visiting and reacquainting themselves with stories of the "good old days".

Two books were compiled as a tribute to our legacy. A book of short concise individual family histories was assembled to document births, marriages, deaths and personal stories. A cookbook preserving favorite family recipes was collected and it still stands today as a "go-to bible" in the kitchens of many family and friends.

The family is proud of Olga's success, adventures and see her enthusiasm and inspiration as a guiding torch for future generations.

My daughters Nadine, Lynda, and her husband Richard attended the reunion. Lynda reminisced about summer holidays with her cousins on the farm.

Some of my happiest memories include spending summer vacations on the Gutiw and Chomyn farms. I recall walking and calling for the cows at 3 o'clock in the afternoon (trying to avoid the cow pies), secretly smoking cigarettes with cousin Mary Jane Gutiw in the abandoned car in the pasture, attempting to milk the cows (I don't think I ever got the hang of it), picking mushrooms, making noodles for chicken noodle soup, playing hide and seek in the yard after it got dark, running to the outhouse in the middle of the night, and having to wake up bright and early in the morning to do chores all over again.

I also recall a specific incident on the Gutiw farm involving my sister, Nadine, and a cow called Eugenia. Eating a meal at the Gutiw farm was a sight to behold: people and food everywhere.

Then I remember walking along the railway track to school in Carpenter, Saskatchewan with cousin Jerry. I remember watching through a crack in the barn wall as Uncle Matt Chomyn and Jerry helped deliver a calf. I remember stooking bales and helping to harvest rape seed. I remember Jerry trying in vain to teach me the difference between wheat, barley and oats, and I'm still not sure how many acres there are in a quarter (or is it the other way around?). I still can't figure out how the rocks come back every year to the fields after we had spent so much time the year before getting rid of them. I cherish these memories and hope that one day my children will be able to experience some of these wonderful times.

I was the first of my ten siblings to leave a marriage. Although I knew in my heart that I had made the right choice, being a single parent was a difficult experience. Women of my generation were resigned to married life, for better or for worse, 'til death do us part. Someone asked me what would have happened if I had stayed married to John and, truthfully I think, as a battered wife, I would be dead by now.

When I arrived in New Westminster as a young 34-year-old mother, I realized that my children needed spiritual, social, and moral nurturing. The best way I knew to provide for them was by associating with the church community.

At Holy Eucharist Ukrainian Catholic Cathedral in New Westminster, I became one of the founding members. I helped preserve and develop the Ukrainian language and culture by conducting Ukrainian lessons through speaking, writing, reading, and singing as well as Easter egg writing, cross-stitch embroidery, and Ukrainian dance.

In 1956, I joined the Ukrainian Catholic Women's League of Canada (UCWLC) New Westminster Branch.

The UCWLC mission statement proclaims that the church aims to:

> Foster a comprehensive understanding of our Ukrainian Catholic religious and cultural heritage;

> Enrich its members' dedication to social justice and spirituality;

> Support its members toward the goal of fulfilling their role in the church and society; and

> Nurture an environment that recognizes the family as the basic unit of society.

This group of committed UCLWC members works diligently to maintain a strong spiritual and cultural identity in the rich fabric of the Canadian experience as well as provide charitable support to organizations in Ukraine. In 1989, after Ukraine gained independence, the economy remained poor, and there was dire need on behalf of orphans and the elderly.

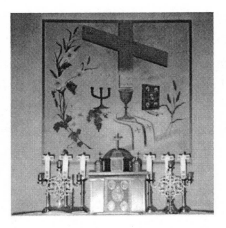

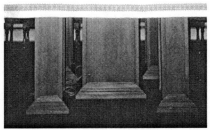

The icon I painted for Holy Eucharist
Cathedral in New Westminster.

In over 50 years of being a UCWLC member, I contributed to the organization, our church, community, children and youth in any way that I could: Branch President (1969), Corresponding Secretary UCWLC Eparchial Executive (1974), UCWLC Eparchial President (1984-86), Vice-President and Chairperson Public Relations (1986-89), and member on numerous other various committees. I helped with fundraising projects, took part in a Candlelight Walk and Ecumenical Prayer vigils at an abortion clinic, and compiled slides and articles regarding our spiritual and cultural traditions in our Eparchy.

In 1969, I painted an 8'x 8' icon for Holy Eucharist cathedral which hung behind the altar on the Sanctuary Wall for many years. A new Eparchy was formed in 1977, and I took on a number of tasks to help build the framework of a new UCWLC Eparchial Executive in B.C.

I was invited to accompany the late Rev. Bishop Jerome Chimy, OSBM and Sister Jerome to Curitiba, Brazil to celebrate three historic religious events. The hospitality of the Ukrainian people in Brazil was overwhelming.

One very sublime encounter with local children made me believe that innocence is bliss. Seven happy youngsters were on their way to grandma's place one calm peaceful Saturday morning. Each carried a bag. As we became more acquainted, I asked one boy what was in his bag. As if on cue, a rooster head popped out of his bag. "Tomorrow we will celebrate my 10th birthday with a delicious dinner," he replied with great anticipation. There have to be many rewards in such a vibrant community as in Curitibo, Brazil.

On one of my later journeys to Europe, I joined a tour to Medjugore, historically the place where the Blessed Virgin Mary appeared to a group of children. During the liturgy, Father Isadore realized there was no spoon available to serve Holy Communion. In my purse, I had a ring of small tools: scissors, file, clippers, and a spoon. We were so thankful that we could continue with the service and receive Holy Communion with my little spoon. It remains now as a relic in the chapel in Medjugore.

In 1988 a celebration of the Millennium of Christianity in Ukraine was held in Rome at the Vatican. Joint Ukrainian church choirs from B.C. and Alberta responded in the Holy Liturgy celebration with His Holiness Pope John Paul II at the Basilica. The most poignant moment was the singing of "The Lord's Prayer" by one of our church choir members. During the pope's visit to Vancouver, I received Holy Eucharist from the hands of Pope John Paul II. It is a precious memory.

In 1984, I co-authored, with my UCWLC colleague, Yaroslava Tatarniuk, *The Ukrainian Traditional and Modern Cuisine Cookbook.* This 140-page cookbook was dedicated in honour of the 40th anniversary of the Ukrainian Catholic Women's League in Canada and the 10th anniversary of the Eparchy of New Westminster. It proved to be very popular and has had four reprints. Sales of the cookbook have raised over $60,000.

Initially the money was to be used to build an eparchial museum, but that was not feasible because the Eparchy had no property or money for a building. Bishop Severian Yakymyshyn then suggested that a contribution be made towards an Iconostas that would be installed in the Holy Eucharist Cathedral in New Westminster. The Iconostas represent the holy icons of the Mother of God and other Saints.

The cookbook committee was proud of its hard work in producing, printing, and distributing hundreds of copies of the cookbook. We were proud to be able to contribute towards the installation of Holy Icons at both our Eparchy and also in Ukraine, especially the icon of the Mother of God, Patroness of our UCWLC organization.

My devotion and dedication to my community have never faltered, and for my 56 years of service I was bestowed with an honorary UCWLC Life Membership. In 2011, I was awarded the Nation Builders Award of the Ukrainian Canadian Congress,

Saskatchewan Provincial Council in appreciation for many years of service in our community.

Several times a year I join other volunteers to make 350–500 dozen pyrogies for church fundraisers. A local newspaper reporter came to watch our production line, and she exclaimed there is power behind a plate of pyrogies. I agree. These tasty morsels have funded many worthwhile projects both here in Canada and in Ukraine.

Ukrainians enjoy a variety of cultural and religious traditions. Besides weddings, celebrations such as Easter are an important part of Ukrainian community life. For Ukrainians, Easter has a great significance because of its specific religious rites, traditional baking, and decorated Easter eggs that have artistic designs of symbolic nature. The decorated Easter eggs are called *pysanky* from the word *pysaty*, which means to write. After the introduction of Christianity, the decorated eggs became a symbol of new spiritual life.

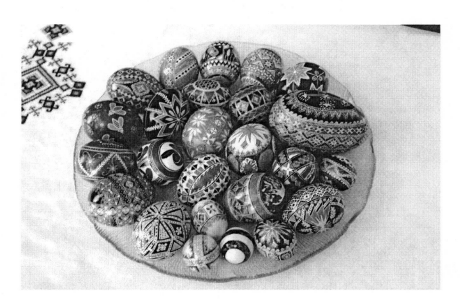

A selection of my decorated Easter eggs. Noris Burdeniuk photo.

The *pysanky* are raw eggs covered with colourful geometric or plant designs symbolizing life, well-being, and abundance. Each Easter egg represents the independence and uniqueness of each human being. Also, it is a mystical metaphor: from its covered space there emerges, as from a mother's womb, a new being that is born. So, too, from the tomb a body is called back to life again. The egg is a strong reminder that only God has the power to give life.

I have been making *pysanky* for many years, and I love how a fragile and commonplace egg can be transformed into a new, beautiful, and unique entity. Young children and youth especially are deeply touched when their Easter egg has been completed. The *pysanky* are a tribute to the feast, a hymn in colour and design, and a fine gift to share with others. Having roots in the pre-Christian Kyivan Rus, they were adapted to Christianity and have been part of the paschal celebrations.

A beautiful tradition maintained in the Ukrainian church tradition is the blessing of food at Easter. *Paska* is the most important Easter food and symbolizes Christ and the resurrection as it represents the bread of eternal life. Decorated with a braided wreath and a cross in the center, it is distinctly in honour of the Resurrection and a reminder of the Eucharistic bread. At Easter, the bread becomes the centerpiece, reverentially placed on a small doily-like altar linen. Christ is the guest of honour at the table.

For Ukrainians, the most beloved and joyful festival is Christmas. Some Ukrainian Christmas customs have historical roots reaching back to the Neolithic era and are connected with the agricultural way of life of our ancestors. After the official introduction of Christianity in Rus-Ukraine in 988 by Prince Volodymyr the Great, many of these folk customs and rites have been properly adapted to the spirit of the Christian religion.

The most important and colourful part of the Christmas tradition and festivities is Christmas Eve (*Sviat Vechir*), which revolves around the twelve-course Lenten supper. This family reunion commemorates the ancestors and the religious observance of Christmas. For the Christmas Eve supper, the table is strewn with a small handful of hay in memory of the Christ Child born in the manger, and spread over it is the best tablecloth adorned with richly decorated embroidery. The central table decoration constitutes a *kolach* (a fancy braided bread). In some parts of Ukraine, one can find just one *kolach* with a candle inserted in the centre, while in others as many as three *kolachi* are placed on top of each other, and the bottom loaf is adorned with small twigs of evergreen. The word *kolach* derives from *kolo* meaning round or circular and it is a symbol of the sun. The centerpiece of three *kolachi* represents the Holy Trinity, while the candle—the Light of the World—symbolizes the star that shone over the stable in Bethlehem.

If a member of the family had died during the year, a place is set for her/him at the table in the belief that the spirit of the deceased unites with the family on that Holy Night. *Sviata Vechera* Holy Supper itself consists of twelve meatless dishes representing the twelve apostles who shared the Last Supper with Jesus Christ. We prepare the dishes with vegetable oil: this custom reflects the omitting of all animal fat.

As mentioned in chapter three, the main and first-served dish is *kutya*, which is whole wheat cooked for many hours and prepared with honey and ground poppy seed. The origin of *kutya* dates back 5000 years when the ancestors of the Ukrainian people first cultivated wheat. This ritual dish has ancient symbolic, religious, and agricultural meanings and represents a continuance of family unity. Wheat, honey, and poppy seeds symbolize the fertility of God's nature; therefore, *kutya* is accepted as a symbol for peace, prosperity, and good health.

After the solemn meal, the family joins in singing carols (*koliady*). The most popular carol is "*Boh Predvichney Narodyvsya*" (God Eternal is Born). At midnight everyone attends the Holy Liturgy at the parish church.

Ukrainian carols *koliady* and *shchedrivky*, sung by the Ukrainian people during Christmas, are generally known because of their unique musical harmony, beauty, and joyful inspiration. Many express agricultural motifs with wishes for good health, happiness, and abundance in the New Year. The main theme of our carols, such as *koliadky*, is strictly religious, glorifying the advent of Jesus Christ as the Saviour of the world. It may be noted that a popular carol in North America, "the Carol of the Bells", is actually a Ukrainian *shchedrivka*, a New Year carol.

As you can see, I love my community and our Ukrainian traditions. My Ukrainian heritage has been a significant contributor to my identity, as have been my Canadian background and my connections to New Westminster and West Vancouver. Heritage of place is like an external inheritance: where you're born and where you live help develop character and enhance self-image. I am grateful for the many friends and lovely celebrations within my community that have enriched my life.

To give back to my community, I taught school for 34 years, and today I sing in two Ukrainian choirs, namely Vancouver St. Mary's church choir and *Svitanok* Folk Chorus. The magic that arises from the joy of music makes singing a healthy pastime. Singing or engaging in any kind of music is healthy for the mind, body, and spirit. The therapeutic power of music boosts our resistance to infections, calms anxiety, and helps us sleep better. It makes me feel great and improves my mood.

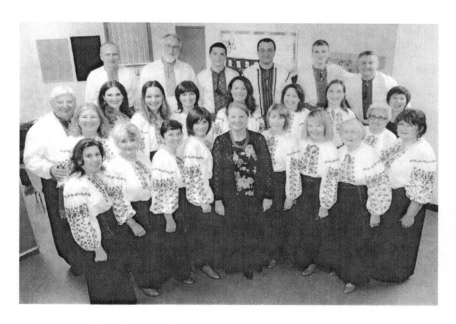

The *Svitanok* Folk Chorus with choir leader
Ann Kvitka Kozak. Photo by Leo Lui.

I thank my Guardian Angel for protecting me, and thank my God for guiding me and sustaining my good health in body, mind, and spirit. Throughout my life, I have recognized that God's love is also a part of my heritage, and I count my blessings every day. Little did I know how much I would need this deep abiding faith as well as my precious community to help me cope during a very dark time in my life.

My elder daughter Nadine would often refer to me as "my mother the jock". She watched me compete a number of times, and I knew that she was as proud of me as I was of her. Nadine followed in my footsteps and became a teacher and taught in Burnaby schools for 20 years. In 1993, she and her partner, John Vendetti, opened a lovely Italian restaurant in Coquitlam called "The Stinking Rose". It was a garlic lover's paradise and featured garlic in all of its fine dishes. A newspaper reporter commented on its fine atmosphere and incomparable cuisine, calling it "Coquitlam's Best Kept Secret". It was a treat to visit their restaurant and to know my daughter had worked so hard on creating its décor, cuisine, and excellent service.

In 1999, my daughter Nadine passed away after a ten-year battle with non-Hodgkins lymphoma. I find it difficult to talk about Nadine's death even to this day. It is against nature for a parent to bury her child.

After Nadine's death, I realized that the only thing I could control was my attitude and mental competence. Life has a way of making you adapt to circumstances that are beyond your control. There is no training program or vitamin that makes you immune to misfortune or circumstances that are beyond your control. I threw myself into my sports, and I maintained a strong connection to my community to cope with the traumatic loss. For several years, I captained a team from St. Mary's Parish in the Cancer Society's Relay for Life, a popular cancer fundraiser. Our parish has raised thousands of dollars and was ranked 6th out of 29 teams in terms of money raised.

Wonderful West Vancouver

When I retired from teaching and moved to West Vancouver, I soon realized that I was fortunate to live in an outstanding vibrant community. The West Vancouver Seniors Centre is a centre of inspiration with over 600 active volunteers who provide leadership, knowledge, and skills to enhance the quality and growth of the centre and its members. According to Jill Lawlor, community recreation manager, "Members learn. Members play. Members inspire". The centre hosts a variety of activities, events, and programs ranging from art classes to snooker, technology classes to quilting bees. The warm and welcoming Garden Side Café weekly offers a variety of healthy hot lunches and dinners.

The West Vancouver Recreation Centre has become my home away from home where I work out in the exercise room and take part in aquafit (aerobics in the water). Fitness experts tell us that for long-range health benefits, it's best to cross-train our bodies by emphasizing aerobics one day, weight training the next, and perhaps yoga on the day after that. Walk on Mondays. Swim on Tuesdays. That is the model that I follow for cardiovascular conditioning, balance, flexibility, and strength training.

If you have never been to a gym, you will soon overcome your intimidation when you enter the gym at the West Vancouver Recreation Centre. Go directly to an attendant who works there; introduce yourself and explain why you have come. He or she needs to know your status: tell them what your intentions are, so they can devise a suitable plan for where you need to start. You will soon become acquainted with the various exercise machines, why this one, why that one, and what you will gain by using it. The attendant will start you off with a routine he or she feels is right for you. Go for it! There you are. That wasn't so bad. The attendants are knowledgeable about how to get you started. They can shepherd you and instruct you as you move along to health and wellness.

Be brave. No inhibitions. They are there to help you. Some day you will thank me for this advice.

I am obsessed with aquasize, a non-stop session of stretching, cardio, and weights that will help you get in shape too. I chose the Aquafit *plus* class. My one-hour aquafit class begins at 7:30 a.m. Mondays, Wednesdays, and Fridays. The class consists of 45 eager, early-rising men and women. It is a terrific place for fitness and fun. Exercising in the water feels differently from exercising on land. It is a unique training medium. Aqua fitness is challenging to do, and it requires concentration and practice. Even to stay suspended, you need to work hard. By using the water effectively you will achieve the right intensity of the exercise. Water pushes back only as hard as you push against it. You realize that the water is so powerful; therefore, adequate strength and endurance are necessary to get the best results from the exercise. Workouts can be as gentle or as hard as you decide to make them. You soon become comfortable in the aquatic environment and begin to enjoy the unique fitness training.

Exercising aerobically in the shallow water makes the heart pound and the lungs fill up with oxygen while focusing on the cardio-respiratory fitness. This boosts energy, reduces stress, and calms the body. As you age, exercise regularly to increase your vitality, endurance, flexibility, and balance—things that tend to decrease with age. Regular aerobic exercise prevents heart disease, lowers blood pressure and cholesterol, controls body weight, and improves cardiovascular fitness. Stroke, depression, osteoporosis, and arthritic patients' reports show they suffer from less pain and disability when they do aquafit exercises. Continually, we keep huffing and puffing, filling our lungs with more oxygen. We become aware of air that we cannot see and seldom think about it. But we breathe about

5000 gallons of air every day, and without it we would survive only a few short minutes. Our muscles and organs need to get that extra oxygen, so we exercise aerobically.

The focus is on cardiovascular fitness, muscular strength, and endurance. The target heart rate for the cardio-respiratory exercise is between 60 and 80% of the maximum heart rate for your age. Maximum heart rate is determined by using the formula 220 minus age x 10 intensity. To achieve these benefits we walk, jog, kick, ski, jump, ski cross country, do rocking horse, and incorporate our jumping jacks while in the water. We use dumbbells and noodles (styrofoam tubes) to improve muscular strength and endurance by overloading the muscle groups continually and rhythmically. We need a strong heart and set of lungs to deliver life-giving oxygen to the muscles. The last group of exercises is for improving balance, something that we can lose as we age.

I am very fond of the Jacuzzi-hot tub. Before I get into the hot tub, I sit on its edge and place my feet against the jets for about 10 minutes to get the soles of my feet energized by this form of reflexology. Experience the great feeling when you place your hands loosely against the jets. I have been able to utilize as many as 3 jets at the same time on various parts of my body. My hands and fingers get energized in the same way.

After a track and field championship, I make a straight dash to the hot tub to calm down my aching muscles. This, I truly believe, is the salvation for my busy body. I love this and have done it for years. With warm-water pool therapy the water temperature should be 90° or warmer. This therapy improves balance, stretches muscles, relieves pressure on the spine, begins to strengthen the muscles in the body, and soothes us physically and emotionally.

After morning aqua fit classes, while I am eating breakfast and reading a newspaper, I find myself dozing off into my porridge because I have worked so hard in the swimming pool.

It is much easier to maintain a positive attitude when we enjoy good health. Meeting my regular aquafit chums three times a week keeps me engaged with other people and helps me to maintain a positive outlook on life. I make a conscious effort to be extroverted and energetic. I believe that optimists have fewer physical and emotional difficulties, enjoy higher energy levels, and are happier and calmer. I am so grateful to have this opportunity for exercise and community. I am also enrolled in the Healthy Aging Study with the B.C. Cancer Agency.

On March 10, 2009 at the Seymour Golf and Country Club more than 90 family, friends and neighbours celebrated my 90 birthday. On the occasion of my birthday, one of my aquafit chums wrote this poem:

So Olga is ninety
Oh how can that be!
She acts like she might be
Fifty one, two or three.
Six in the morning she's sure to be up,
Rarin' to go just like a young pup.
She scoots out the back of her house it's been found,
Where the "Fountain of Youth"
bubbles up through the ground.
There she gargles and brushes and takes a good sip
Then just to be sure she partakes in a dip.
Next it's off to a track, a game or a meet
To break a few records, accomplish some feat.

Olga. The O.K. Way to a Healthy, Happy Life.

It's really embarrassing here in the pool,
She makes us feel lazy (with cause as a rule)
She shows us all up with the flick of a wrist,
To us it's all work— to her mill, it's just grist.
It's become quite annoying—she's medal-some too—
Big gold ones on ribbons of red and of blue.
But enough of this fooling it's all said in jest
And we want her to know that she's simply the best.
We've all agreed—without one nay-sayer
That she'll always be our "most valuable player".
Happy Birthday, Olga!

June MacDonald
Aquafit *Plus* Club
West Vancouver Aquatic Centre

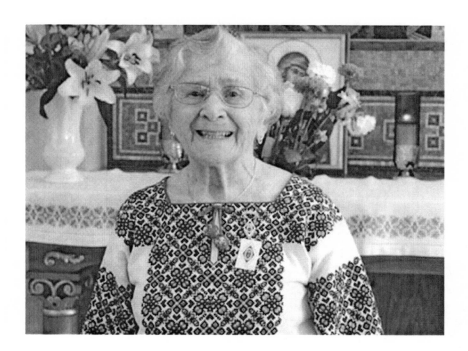

I truly believe that to maintain a healthy lifestyle and a cheerful disposition you must seek out the company of others, be eager to meet people, and to establish new friendships.

Camaraderie is the key to success when dealing with all of the sadness, frustration, and stress that life can bring. Research has shown that the healthiest people who live the longest enjoy the company of the most friends. People around the world, who live the longest usually have wide social networks as well as a sense of purpose. A connection to others helps to combat unhealthy self-absorption.

A lack of connectivity may be the No. 1 problem in the modern world. People sit glued to their TVs watching mindless programs for hours, or sit at their computers communicating with people living thousands of miles away, but they can't or won't go for a walk around the block. Just saying you're going to achieve a goal or fulfill a promise is not enough; you actually have to get up and follow through. Do it for yourself because you're worth it. And remember, when you have something to offer and contribute to your community and neighbourhood, everyone profits from the effort.

Helping the Scientific Community
My First Visit to McGill University

It all started in Lahti, Finland the year I turned 90. The World Masters Athletics Championships were held July 27–August 11, 2009, where some 10,000 athletes aged 35 to 100 years participated.

Dr. Tanja Taivassalo had come to Finland to cheer on her 70-year-old father who was running in his first marathon. As a runner herself, she was astonished to see me, this 90-year-old athlete, run fast enough that the wind was gently blowing my hair back. When she saw me doing my thing and go on to win eight World Records, she became curious both personally and professionally. She invited me to McGill University for study and research. Does one say "no"? Of course not. Besides, no one could be more curious than I. At the age of 90, why did I still have the energy and stamina that I had as a young 50-year-old? Where was my strength and energy coming from? It was a mystery even to me.

Dr. Taivassalo is an associate professor at McGill University's Department of Kinesiology and Physical Education. She explained to me that her area of research is the mitochondria, the power source of the body's cells involved in healing and growth. Her subjects are usually young people who suffer from a genetic disease that makes them so weak they can hardly walk around the block. She explained that some researchers see aging as a kind of mitochondrial disease, eventually robbing the aging population of endurance, strength, and function. Was there a way to keep those energy-producing mitochondria from shrinking as we age? Perhaps by studying me, she could help others.

Her research partner and husband, Dr. Russell Hepple, is an associate professor in the Department of Kinesiology, Physical Education, and the Department of Medicine (Critical Care Division). Dr. Hepple studies muscle fibers, and he hoped that what he would find in me might challenge the current wisdom that all old people will inevitably lose valuable muscle fibers as they age.

Over several days, I gave my body over to medical science, and I allowed them to test me for muscle mass, strength, and endurance. They actually had to get special permission to test someone who was over 85 years of age.

Day 1: Dr. Hepple delivered a 1 ½ hour lecture entitled "Exercise Pathophysiology — Physiology of Aging". We then proceeded to the Montreal Chest Hospital where lung and heart ECG rhythm-function testing was done. The doctor then scheduled me for a body composition scan (bone density and maximal muscle strength) to take place after lunch.

That evening at the Finnish Lutheran Church, Canadian Friends of Finland, Dr. Taivassalo led a presentation on physiology, and I spoke about my athletic career and demonstrated my finger and sponge ball exercises. (You will learn these wonderful exercises in the next chapter.)

Day 2: At the Montreal Chest Hospital, I underwent exhausting testing on the treadmill for peak aerobic exercise capacity. Dr. Hepple worked me to my fullest potential until I could not continue. In the transparent plastic cubicle (similar to a telephone booth), my chest function was monitored by specific deep breathing through a mouthpiece, which checked my heart rate and blood pressure. Blood sampling was done concurrently by a study physician to ensure that the amount of blood that was withdrawn in intervals was not going to affect my health.

The day after the treadmill test, I was taken to the free-weight gym at McGill University. I lay down at the bench press, and Dr. Hepple and the other researchers started adding weights to the ends of the bar. Although I am right-handed, I discovered that I am quite a bit stronger on my left-side. By the time I was on the sixth rep of my bench presses, it was so quiet in the gym you could hear a pin drop! The young men in the gym stopped exercising, and they were staring at someone who could have been their grandmother bench press 60 pounds without too much effort.

Day 3: My first assignment was to address a class of 100 under-graduate students enrolled in the Exercise Pathophysiology and Aging Program. These young minds knew that many elderly individuals do not engage in any sort of exercise or physical activity as different systems in the body decline in function. I spoke about my experiences in track and field, including my times and distances for the various events, the types and levels of competitions, what endurance hurdles I have and will continue to face, my training routine, and the times and distances between my first place results and the results of the second place finishers.

The doctor performed a muscle biopsy for specific study on muscle fiber type, function and ability to regenerate. Dr. Horme Morais injected my left thigh with a freezing solution, and when it took hold he made a small scalpel incision in my quad. The first muscle sample was not great, and I could see Dr. Taivassalo and Dr. Hepple try to hide their disappointment. But Dr. Morais went a little deeper and, eventually, plucked out two beautiful pieces of raw, red muscle each about the size of a pea. Someone said it looked like sushi, which made me laugh because sushi is a food I never, ever eat and now definitely will never try! They froze the muscle sample in liquid nitrogen, and a grad student rushed the specimen to a lab at the University of Montreal.

They analyzed a biopsy of three pieces of my muscle, and a technician declared that, "This is the healthiest muscle I have seen in my life. This muscle could belong to an 18-year-old!" Imagine, 91-year-old muscle! I presented him with one of my gold medals.

This was the last day of testing. What an experience to be involved in this study. In the end, the researchers determined the following: "Aerobic capacity is very good and it is equivalent to a

60-year-old. As well, Olga has exceptional muscle fibers that allow her to excel in power sports".

Power sports! Before the age of 77, I didn't know what that term meant. I was never a serious jock as a young girl, and later on I was too busy teaching and raising my children to take part in any sports. But when I discovered track and field in my late 70s, I experienced a sense of joy I had not felt in a very long time. My athletic persona had percolated below the surface most of my life, certainly during those years back in Saskatchewan, as a girl and a teacher, where baseball and walking had kept me in shape, but I never expected to become an athlete whose abilities warranted scientific investigation, especially in my late 70s. The athlete in me had risen to the surface, and I greeted her with open arms.

During all the testing, the doctors had made an interesting discovery. Scientists say fast-twitch muscle fibres are essential in sports such as sprinting, which requires short-duration explosive movement. I seem to have some similar muscle fibre for sprinting because I have world records in 200m, 400m, 800m, but not in 100m. Likely not quite that fast a twitch for 100m.

According to Dilson Rassier, a muscle physiology expert and associate professor in the Department of Kinesiology and Physical Education at McGill University, fast-twitch muscle fibres are blessed with good genetics. Fast-twitch muscles contract and fatigue quickly. They're used primarily for short duration, highly explosive movements like sprinting, throwing, and jumping. I do all that in my competitions, and I don't mind that I don't twitch fast enough for 100m: for me, my jumping and throwing events are twitching fast enough. I thank my mom and dad and, of course, God for blessing me so abundantly.

The following is from the paper documenting the experiments written by Dr. Taivassalo and her research team.

"The benefits and results from this Study and Research may provide the medical community (neurologists, cardiologists and pulmonary doctors) with valuable information to better diagnose future patients presenting with similar symptoms and exaggerated cardiovascular and ventilator exercise responses. Furthermore, it will provide the scientific community with a better understanding of regulatory mechanisms within muscles that link oxygen delivery to utilization. This study may also provide the medical community with information about ways to design exercise training protocols to improve muscle mitochondrial function and normalize the exaggerated responses in patients with muscle disease or elderly individuals" (Taivassalo et al, 2010).

My Second Visit to McGill Study and Research

I was very happy to be of use to the McGill research community, and I agreed to return to Montreal for a follow-up session. Since they lacked my other siblings to compare their results, they could gain important data by comparing results from the 2010 experience.

During the second week in October 2012, the Kinesiology Department at McGill University was celebrating its 100th anniversary with the theme "Actively Moving Forward".

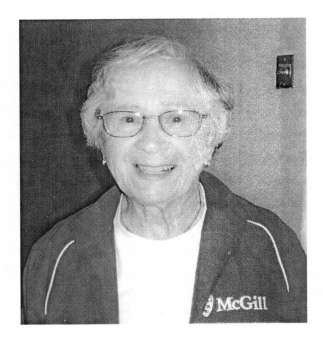

Proudly wearing my McGill jacket.

Day 1: Dr. Taivassalo invited me to attend the anniversary banquet. I was honoured for being "an exemplary role model". The evening's guest speaker and McGill alumni, Mike Babcock, shared with us how it felt to win an Olympic Gold Medal as coach of the Canadian hockey team at the Vancouver 2010 Winter Olympics.

Day 2: Early Sunday morning, my assignment was to use the starting pistol to start the marathon. With the gun nowhere to be found I was given a foghorn instead.

Day 3: On Monday October 15, I received the schedule for the rest of the week. It resembled the schedule for my first visit in 2010; however, more comprehensive testing was anticipated. There would not be two sets of results to compare.

As we age, heart, lung, and muscle function decline in people, especially for those in their 60s and 70s; consequently, a need exists to focus on people in their 80s and 90s and to study their exercise response.

During this second visit, I underwent an ECG as I rode a stationary bike as hard as I could. They measured the cardiac output which gauged how much my heart had to pump. They also did a full body composition scan, using a DEXA machine, which took an accurate snapshot of how much bone, muscle, and fat my body contains.

My muscle and brain were scanned with an MRI machine. They took blood samples to look for, among other things, markers of inflammation, which happens when the body is trying to repair itself, and for chemicals like BDNF, a secreted protein that helps protect and grow the brain.

This was definitely a more comprehensive testing regime than in 2010 and also more exhausting and challenging. They tabled the results of the VO2 kinetics, VO2 peak and Quad biodex and biopsy tests. For me, the hardest and most interesting test was the cognitive assessment test. It was a rush reflection of somewhat similar tests I had taken in my 30s. I struggled and persisted and survived. In the tester's estimation, they may not have been good results. If I had more time to reflect and get adjusted, then I might have done better, but these tests were done instantaneously. A test is a test with criteria.

In 2010, I was the sole subject of the testing, but this time I had company. Also participating in the study were Christa Bortignon (75 years of age) from West Vancouver, B.C., Colin Field, and Arthur Kimber (both 76 years of age), two athletes from England who Dr. Taivassalo had recruited at the World Indoor Championships in Jyvaskyla, Finland.

It was interesting and exciting to meet Arthur and Colin. They were both in great spirits while undergoing testing. I have known Christa for some time now, and she is a great athlete and champion in all dimensions.

All of us considered ourselves quite privileged to have been invited to McGill University for this study and research. I look forward to a third invitation when I have been requested to return to McGill to compare results from 2010 and 2012 and from those still to be gained in 2014.

My Brain and the Beckman Institute

In somewhat the same way that Dr. Tanja Taivassalo and Dr. Russ Hepple at McGill University were peeking into my muscles, Dr. Arthur Kramer soon would be peeking into my brain. Writer Bruce Grierson needed to add some specific results from MRI and behavior tests to his book entitled *What Makes Olga Run*. Arrangements were made with Dr. Kramer, director of the Beckman Institute at the University of Illinois.

On July 22, 2012, Bruce and I left for Illinois for some cognitive testing. Bruce prearranged the trip so that we could enjoy a little sight-seeing in Chicago, surely one of the world's greatest cities. We settled at the grand old Chicago Hilton and then went off to explore the city. We took a boat tour down the Chicago River, toured the Art Institute of Chicago, wandered the streets, and enjoyed great meals.

The University of Illinois is an impressive place in a small charming university town called Champaign. It is home to the National Centre for Supercomputing that happens to be right next door to the Beckman Clinic, home of North America's most cutting-edge work in cognitive science.

Dr. Art Kramer is an energetic, former college athlete who heads up the research facility that is home to a couple of hundred faculty and grad students from some three dozen countries. Dr. Kramer had read Bruce's story in *The New York Times*, and he was interested to meet me and to see what kind of shape my brain was in. The Beckman Institute was the perfect place to find out.

I was introduced to some very nice and smart grad students including doctoral student Laura Chaddock, who had arranged our visit. I embarked on a full day of testing that started at the Biomedical Imaging Center where I underwent brain scans in the MRI machine. They told me I am now the oldest patient in their database!

I did something called a "flanker task", which involved identifying changes in a pattern. While my brain did that work, technicians were looking at movements of blood flow in my brain. They were also interested in my response speed. The brain's processing speed generally slows down as we age. These tests were so peaceful and calm that I almost fell asleep. Later, one of the technicians said that my brain looked like the brains of some of the fifty-year-olds she had seen.

After a nice lunch at an Italian restaurant across town, we were driven to the Illinois Simulator Laboratory. There I undertook something called the "Street-crossing Experiment". In a virtual reality environment, my ability to "multi-task" would be tested. Multi-tasking means paying attention to more than one thing at a time, and it is an ability that usually declines with age.

A street scene was projected on a big screen in front and to the sides of me, and as I walked on a treadmill I seemed to be moving through that street scene. I wore headphones so I could hear the instructions from the tester. The idea was to cross the street without being hit by a car. But as I was concentrating on the traffic, I was being distracted by questions coming in my ear from the tester. Could I answer the questions and still safely navigate my way across the road?

It felt like I was jay-walking through non-stop constant traffic of moving cars going in opposite directions at different intervals. It was scary: my wits were constantly disrupted but desperately needed; my life and safety were at stake.

I felt desperate. I demanded that the tester shut up because she was not helping me but was disrupting my concentration in this hectic situation. She did not hesitate for a moment, and she continued to interrupt right up to the end of this grueling test. It was pretty tiring, and by the end of the experience I was sweating profusely. When the results came in, I had scored 98%.

Then it was back to the Beckman Institute and the Lifelong Brain & Cognition Lab for behavioural and memory testing. A handsome and genial young tester named Andrew put me through my paces there. I had to recall a sequence of random numbers. I had to re-tell the story that I had just heard, recalling as many details as I could.

To test my spatial ability, I had to rotate patterns in my mind. As this was a timed test, I was off my spatial ability, and performed inadequately. Later on in the next sequence of testing, I began to relax and enjoy the tests, and I picked up quickly. I believe my mark was quite low in this behavioural testing. I will have to find out my score in Bruce's book.

Later on that evening, I was treated to a well-earned dinner at a local restaurant with Dr. Kramer and his wife, Laura, and

Bruce. When we arrived back in Vancouver, we learned that Laura was now Dr. Laura Chaddock. Congratulations! She deserved the honours.

While we awaited the testing, Dr. Kramer and Laura asked if they could write an academic paper about me. I feel that such tests can provide the scientific community much needed information and material that can be beneficial into the research of aging. I thank Dr. Art Kramer and his entire staff for being so kind, accommodating, supportive and, above all, professional. After the results from all of the focused games on memory logic, speed, visuals, and concentration were analyzed, the whole experience will be recorded precisely in *What Makes Olga Run*. I can't wait to read Bruce's book!

My message is: motivate yourself and become active. Exercise your body to improve your health and enjoy a happy, healthy lifestyle. Prevention is your best strategy for a strong and healthy cardiovascular system. "Use it or lose it!"

Your homework assignment:

Never miss an opportunity to be of service to someone or something. Search out organizations that could use your help.

Today, find ways of letting go of any fears that may be holding you back from connecting to new people, places, and things.

Appreciate all of the blessings in life, and share your grateful vitality with others. Allow only positive thoughts and feelings to fill your heart and your mind.

Be happy when you go for your daily walk. Smile. Breathe. Go for a swim. Go to the gym. You don't need to do it every day. But go! You may want to alternate your routine for variety.

Play and listen to your favorite music. Dancing is also a great sport in many ways. Action, laughter, music, and camaraderie will enrich your life.

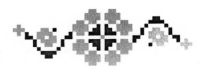

The children were lined up in the cafeteria of a Catholic elementary school for lunch. At the head of the table was a large pile of apples. The nun made a note, and posted on the apple tray: 'Take only one. God is watching'.

Moving further along the lunch line, at the other end of the table was a large pile of chocolate chip cookies.

A child had written a note, 'Take all you want. God is watching the apples'.

Seven
Exercise for a Healthy, Happy OK Lifestyle

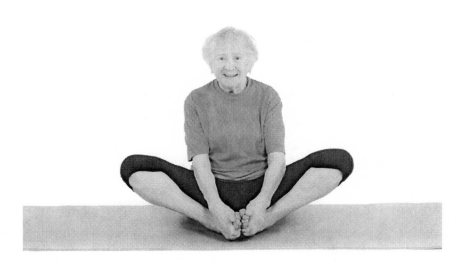

To limber up your groin area and stabilize tension, use
the following ingredients: Persistence is a big fancy
word for "never giving up". Determination is just another
way of saying "no ifs, buts or maybes". Courage is about
"having the guts to do what needs to be done".

Lesson: According to Webster's Dictionary, exercise means a bodily exertion for the sake of developing and maintaining physical fitness. In my experience, it is *the* key to staying young. I am proof that if you diligently follow an exercise program it will add life to your years and years to your life, prevent illness, and help you manage the symptoms of aging. My exercises are practical, challenging, and athletic. The body is strengthened, the mind is alert, and the spirit is free.

"Aging is a new stage of opportunity and strength."
— *Betty Friedan*

All the photos in this exercise chapter
were provided by Cindy Goodman.

"It is impossible to over-estimate the benefits of exercise," according to Dr. Art Hister, a Vancouver family physician and author of numerous health books. "The most important thing we can do to increase our chances of living longer and staying healthy begins with an E, and it's not Eat. Our bodies may need proteins, carbs, vitamins and minerals but oxygen is the most important nutrient we need for every cell of our bodies and we can get that through daily Exercise." As you can see, this well-known doctor believes exercise is the best medicine for successful, healthy aging.

I started to put together my exercise program, *The O.K. Way to a Healthy, Happy Life* about ten years ago when I was some 80 years old. I want to share this program with you because I believe it has helped me achieve the level of good health and physical fitness that I enjoy today.

Some exercise ideas became obvious to me as I received information from different sports' therapists at international track and field competitions. These experts confirmed that vigorous exercise is needed to bring the maximum amount of oxygen into all the cells of the body. Religiously, I work out 3 times a week and alternate days with an aerobic aquafit class. My stretching exercises take place three nights a week in bed. On Sundays, I take a break from exercise, and I attend church to give thanks for my blessings of a healthy body, mind and spirit.

My exercises are practical, challenging, and athletic. I am proof that if you diligently follow an exercise program, it will add life to your years and years to your life.

I realized that a healthy body increases the chance for a longer life, and a healthy mind almost certainly guarantees a more satisfying one. Our thoughts become our words, our words become our actions, our actions become our habits, and our habits become our character. A sound, healthy mind is found in a sound, healthy body.

When strong, invasive thoughts, such as fear or anger come to mind, deep breathing will clear them away. In this way, you can build your mental muscle. Oxygen must be provided to each cell in the body. During my deep breathing exercises, I count from 1 to 4 with each inhalation to fill the lungs with air and 5 to 10 with each exhalation to clear stale air from the lungs. Using this rhythmic technique, I experience less fatigue and exhaustion and, of course, better results in my athletics. I believe that the mental muscle gets built with enough strength to help me in any difficult situation, whether at competitions, at home, or with friends and loved ones. Most of all I become better able to avoid negative emotions like fear and anger and other stresses that make us less than the best we can be.

In the following pages I will demonstrate my personal exercise program.

Stretching

Reflexology— feet

Yoga

Deep Breathing

Facial Massage

Reflexology—hands

Body Massage

Sitting Position

Kneeling Position

Splits

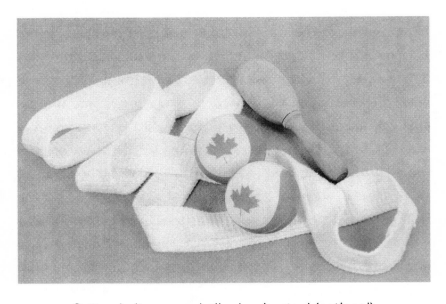

Cotton belt, sponge balls, darning tool (optional).

The materials you will need for my fitness program:

Exercise mat or large towel
2 Sponge Balls (found in dollar store)
Cotton belt
Blunt tool (i.e., darning tool, optional)
Reflexology Chart

I incorporate the activities of **stretching, massage, reflexology, yoga, the use of sponge balls, and a tie belt** into my routine program. I will give a brief description of each of these activities, and I will illustrate how and why I do each exercise. I hope you will benefit from and enjoy the exercises. I use two balls because I use both hands at the same time.

Very Important: Always check with your doctor before starting any exercise program for the first time. Stop working out immediately if you experience any of the following:

Difficulty breathing
Chest pain
Fever
Extreme pain
Feeling too hot
Nausea
Numbness in any body part
Throbbing headache
Dizziness or a feeling the room is spinning

STRETCHING

If you carefully watch a dog or a cat, see how they stretch every day, especially first thing in the morning. We should follow the example of our furry friends. Our modern lifestyle contributes to our muscular tension and stiffness, especially as we age. I believe that these stretching exercises can heal any tired and hurt muscle tissue quickly, and they always bring me back to a calm, healthy state. Also, I believe that cramps may be prevented by exercising and massaging regularly. Regular exercise and massage can have the effect of reducing painful spasms and areas of muscular tightness.

Bob Anderson introduced me to The Basic Program 5 stretching exercises, a program he developed thirty years ago, and I incorporated some of his excellent stretching exercises into my personal health program. Throughout this portion of *The O.K. Way to a Healthy, Happy Life*, you will learn how muscles are continually strengthened in the various exercises. Over the years, I have added and extended ideas to my program to maintain vitality and good health in the whole body.

Stretching is not stressful; you will find it peaceful and relaxing. I stretch frequently and exercise regularly. Each one of us is a unique physical and mental being with our own comfortable and enjoyable ways. We are all different in strength, endurance, flexibility, and temperament. The body's capacity for recovery from serious illness is phenomenal. All of us have this amazingly miraculous capacity for regaining health. Regular stretching will relax your mind and tune-up your unique body. Concentrate on the area being stretched. Deep breathing should be slow, rhythmical, and controlled to develop lung fitness.

Your muscles stretch more easily when your body is properly hydrated. Drink plenty of water, at least 8 glasses a day. Relaxed stretches help your body to function more naturally and to help you sleep soundly. Take your time, stretch with control, and breathe deeply.

As we get older, we go through periods of inactivity and then activity again. We cause stress and strain on the knees, lower legs, ankles, and arches. If you have had knee problems, be careful bending the knees: do it slowly and under control. If there is any pain, discontinue the stretch. The same holds true for any other reasons. It is better to under stretch than to over stretch. Always be at a point where you can stretch further and never at a point where you have gone as far as you can go.

Learn to listen to your body. If the stretch builds and you feel pain, your body is trying to let you know that something is wrong, that there is a problem. If this happens, ease off gradually until the stretch feels right. Connect with your body.

I believe that stationary exercises are more beneficial than ballistic ones. No jerking or bouncing. Therefore, I hold most poses for approximately 30 seconds. This has helped me to develop my balance, strength, and stability. In fact, I continually work on maintaining my flexibility and balance. I never sit down to dress, and I remain standing to pull on my socks and put on my pants.

First of all, find a place to exercise that is convenient for you and make it part of your regular routine. Believe it or not, the best time for me to do my stretching exercises is about 2 a.m. After nature calls me to the bathroom, and I am unable to fall asleep again, rather than suffer with insomnia and get up to paint my kitchen or rearrange my spice drawer, I do my exercises in bed. Over the years, every week on Tuesdays, Thursdays, and Saturdays my body has become programmed for these exercises.

These stretching exercises can take 1½ hours for me to complete. Afterwards, I easily fall asleep again, benefit from 4 to 5 more hours of peaceful sleep, and I wake up refreshed at 9 or 10 a.m. Without a doubt, these nighttime exercises have helped to balance my body and mind. I will demonstrate the exercises starting on the right side of my body and then follow on the left side. Stretching is a natural way to reduce aging. Hold each stretch for at least 30 seconds. Make sure that each stretch is felt in your muscles and not your joints. Do not jerk or bounce. Slow down. Work slowly. Have control. No cheating! Focus on holding each stretch during inhalation and on increasing the stretch and releasing tension with each exhalation. A regular, moderate stretching exercise improves your heart and lung fitness and lowers blood pressure. Therefore, you will undoubtedly enjoy a healthier body.

Remember. Listen to your body, and don't do anything that causes pain. Release from each stretch slowly and easily. Here we go!

Exercises To Prevent Illness And Help Manage Symptoms Of Aging

Elongated Stretch

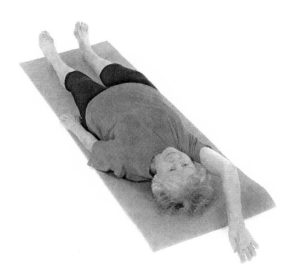

Realign your spine and energize the back muscles. This is a great stretch to do first thing in the morning while still in bed.

Stretch your arms, shoulders, abdominals as well as muscles of the rib cage and legs.

- Lie flat on your back
- Right arm and right leg together reach and pull overhead
- Left leg and arm together push and pull in opposite direction
- Stretch for 30 seconds
- Change direction and stretch for 30 seconds

- With both arms overhead and legs straight pull and stretch in opposite direction for 30 seconds while toes point 15 seconds and flex for 15 seconds

Continually and gently pull in your abdominal muscles to make the middle of your body feel thin. This really feels good! Enjoy the stretch in the shoulder blades.

- Bring hands toward the neck below the ears
- Keep elbows out and down
- Squeeze shoulder blades together; count 30 seconds

Stretches For Abdominal And Back Muscles

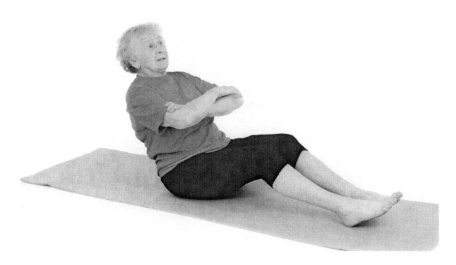

Tighten your pelvic floor muscles, which support the bladder, uterus, small intestine and rectum. This is called a Kegel exercise, and it helps tone and strengthen the pelvic floor muscles. It can help prevent incontinence. This stretch relieves muscular low back pain and tension in the upper back, shoulders, and neck. It tightens the thighs, buttocks and lower abdominal muscles.

- Lie flat on your back with feet front forward
- Bring your body upward leading with your arms to a half-sitting position
- Look ahead
- Hold and count 20 to 30 seconds; relax 2 to 3 seconds
- Repeat this exercise 3 times

Stretch The Calf And Buttocks

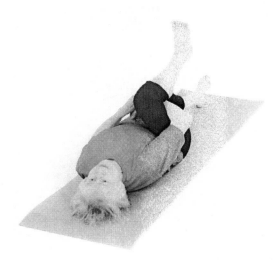

Hold onto the back of the leg to create this stretch.

- Lie flat on your back with legs straight
- Get back of head pressed to the mat
- With both arms pull the right knee toward your chest and hold tightly while rotating the ankle for 30 seconds, 15 clockwise and 15 counterclockwise
- Repeat exercise and alternate with the left knee and rotate ankle for 30 seconds

This rotary motion helps to gently stretch out tight calf, buttocks, and hamstrings and prevents leg cramps.

You may use a foam support under the head. Most seniors have a rounded back that makes it hard to get the back of the head down properly without the support. Only stretch as far as comfortable.

Exercise The Toes

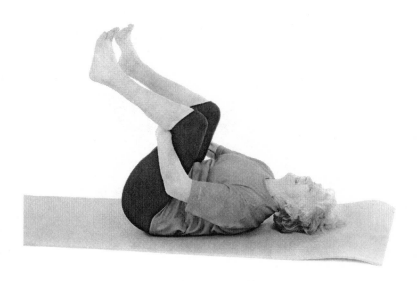

This exercise is meditative for the soul and relaxes the mind. This helps to stretch and strengthen the toes, the bottom of your feet (plantar fascia), and relax the calf muscles.

- With both arms pull both knees to the chest
- Stretch the toes by separating and pulling them apart and outward
- Hold firmly for 30 seconds

My mind seems to wander off and tends to relax as I concentrate on how the toes send energy to my body.

Relaxing Stretches For Your Back, Groin, Hamstrings And Hands

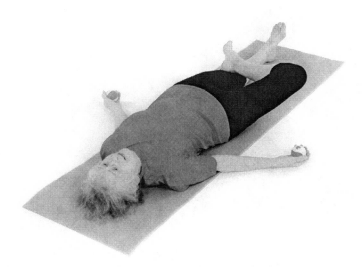

This stretch helps to maintain balance in the body. Crucial for preventing falls. For this excellent leg stretch I use sponge balls to enhance and increase benefits. Sponge balls improve flexibility and circulation of blood and energy in your fingers, wrists, hands, and arms.

- Place right ankle comfortably above the left knee; gently push the bent knee toward the floor
- Hold a sponge ball in each hand and squeeze slowly in a regular sequence for 30 seconds
- Repeat the same exercise with your left ankle above the right knee; push left knee toward the floor and squeeze the balls for 30 seconds

Discipline and determination. Don't cheat. Enjoy the benefits.

Relaxing Stretches For Back, Groin, Hamstrings And Hands

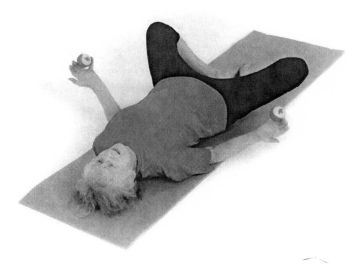

Concentrate as you do these exercises.

- With your knees bent outward bring the soles of your feet together close to your buttocks, to relax these stretches for the back, groin, and hamstrings

- In each hand place a sponge ball comfortably and securely between the baby and ring fingers

- Slowly close the fist all the way while squeezing the balls

- Hold; relax

- Slowly close fists and relax 5 or 10 times

- Move balls to next two fingers and continue exercise, ending with thumb and forefinger

Sponge balls improve circulation in the fingers, hand, wrists, and arms (See the following pages for instructions)

I Will Now Explain How To Use Sponge Balls Between The Fingers

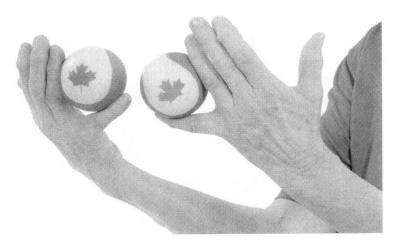

I had never before seen or heard about this type of ball and finger exercise. I wholeheartedly believe in it and highly recommend it. It certainly has helped me. Persist and persevere.

- Comfortably place a sponge ball between baby and ring fingers in each hand and close and open fist slowly 5 or 10 times
- Next place the balls between the ring and middle fingers and again close and open fist slowly 5 or 10 times
- Do the same between the next two fingers and the last two fingers, between the forefinger and the thumb closing and opening fists slowly 5 or 10 times in each hand; don't forget the thumbs

How does this exercise feel now? How are your fingers? You will be amazed how beneficial this exercise can be.

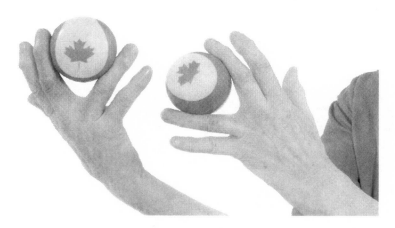

These exercises with foam sponge balls between the fingers have helped me greatly. Several years ago, during cold weather, my fingertips often would turn white, become numb, and hurt. Inventing this exercise with the sponge balls between my fingers has cured my fingertip pain by increasing the energy flow and blood circulation in my fingers, hands, wrists, and arms. It is amazing when you realize that there are 4,000 nerve endings in our hands.

Repetitive motion of the hands when you open and close your hands holding sponge balls may slow down the progression of osteoarthritis, carpal tunnel, tendonitis, and tennis elbow. Sponge balls strengthen the muscles in your hands and wrists, and increase flexibility in the muscles, stimulating the blood and energy circulation. This exercise may be done safely at any age, anywhere, and at any time. Choose sponge balls that fit comfortably in your hand.

Caution: The primary danger of using a sponge ball is overuse. Overuse injuries can occur in the hands and wrists from excessive contraction of the muscles; therefore, I recommend that you use sponge balls in moderation.

Stretch The Quadriceps

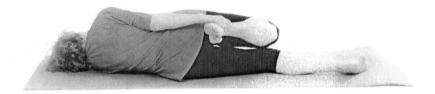

Do not force this stretch if you have any knee pain or discomfort. If your quadriceps say "ouch", simply ease up and try it again.

- Lie straight on your left side, with your spine in a neutral position, pelvis perpendicular to the floor.
- With your right hand reach behind you to hold onto your right foot between toes and ankle joint
- Pull your heel toward the right buttock Keep your knees together
- Push your hips forward to stretch the quadriceps. Hold for 30 seconds
- Repeat the other leg

Exercise For Strengthening Outer Thigh Muscles

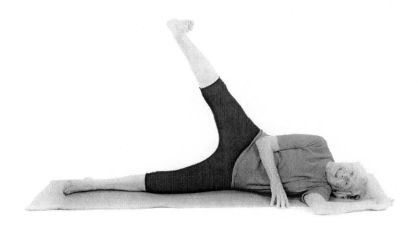

These exercises will help to develop strong muscles for good balance. If your neck is uncomfortable, place a rolled towel under your head.

- Lie straight on left side with your spine in a neutral position, pelvis perpendicular to the floor
- Raise right leg straight from hip, upward as high as possible; try for 90 ° angle
- Raise right leg up and down 30 times
- Repeat exercise on right side, raising left leg straight from your hip up as high as possible
- Raise left leg up and down 30 times

I believe these last two exercises will help to strengthen the leg muscles and help to improve your balance to avoid falling and breaking a bone. As well, you will maintain a strong walking posture. No chicken steps for you or me!

REFLEXOLOGY

I do self-reflexology on my body three times a week during the OK Way Exercises. This zone therapy dates back to ancient Egypt. A particular zone of the foot or hand corresponds to another part of the body, and involves finger and thumb pressure on the feet, hand and, sometimes, the ear. The feet, in particular, provide a map of the entire body, with various parts of the sole connecting to various organs, glands, and limbs.

Those who are unfamiliar with this simple but effective health modality might wonder out loud: who has a liver, a kidney, or a brain in their foot? Yet by massaging different parts of the foot you can stimulate and treat the whole body, the whole person, and not just the symptoms of the disease. The pressure stimulates the flow of energy through the body so that healing can take place naturally.

Reflexology releases blocked energy in the energy pathways of the body. These 12 pathways connect to all the organs and glands, and culminate in the feet as well as the hands. In order to be healthy, these energy pathways must not remain blocked. Reflexology reduces stress (a major contributing factor to disease), enhances the body's ability to heal itself, and balances both body and soul. Research shows that a single reflexology session can create relaxation, reduce anxiety, diminish pain, improve blood flow, and decrease high blood pressure.

Reflexology is used to treat many conditions and illnesses including digestive and circulatory disorders, migraine, back pain, and stress related diseases.

Carefully study the reflexology charts that I have included in this book to see where the pressure points in your hands and feet correspond to different organs, glands, and tissues in your body. Reflexology charts may vary slightly, since reflexology is an unregulated health treatment and, although some say it is not very scientific, somehow it works for me and for countless others.

If you are unsure how to do self-reflexology, consider visiting a trained reflexologist to see how it is performed and to experience the correct pressure to apply.

Whether using a blunt object (I use an old-fashioned darning tool) or your fingers and thumb, apply fine deep pressure of approximately 10 to 15 lbs. of force to appropriate reflex points. This may/can send a surge of energy in the energy pathways to the corresponding areas. Apply pressure for as long and with as much force as you feel comfortable. Reflexology will release blocked energy, open the channels, relieve pain and tension, restore vitality, stimulate organs and glands, and encourage the natural healing process.

Discipline is of the utmost importance in doing reflexology well. Reflexology creates a satisfying sensation on the pressure points for me as I gently move my toes, and I pulsate on the pressure point reflex.

Reflexology is suitable for:

> Acute and chronic conditions
> Sleep disorders
> Stress related conditions
> Children and adults
> Sports injuries
> Prevention therapy

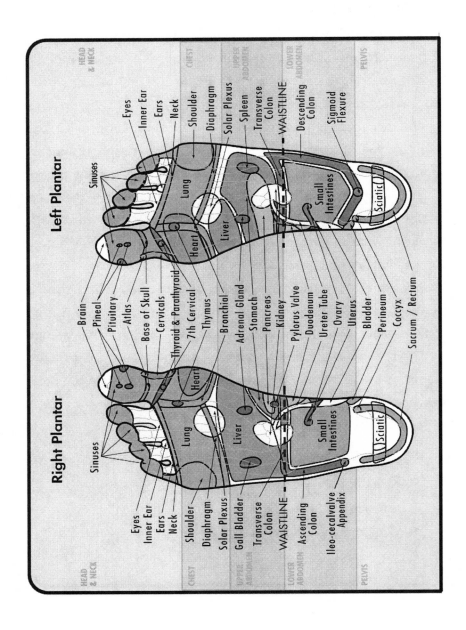

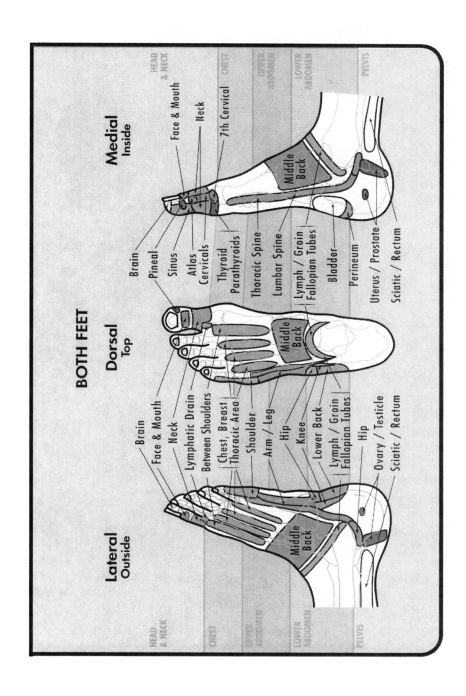

Foot Reflexology

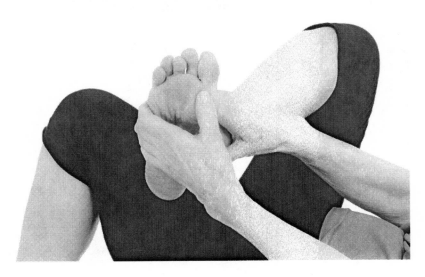

Use the left thumb on the sole of your right foot and your whole right hand on the front of your foot.

Apply deep pressure of approximately 10 to 15 lbs. of force to each reflex point on the sole of your foot. All the reflexes in the foot when correctly stimulated will induce relaxation and relieve stress and tension in the corresponding glands, organs, and other areas of the body.

- Lie on your back and place your right leg over the left thigh above the knee
- With the left thumb begin pressing on the right foot starting just under the big toe; count 10 seconds
- Move your thumb across the foot in a row under the toes pressing on not less than 5 reflex points; count 10 seconds on each point

- Move down slightly and work in the same manner in the opposite direction across the foot

- You should move directions at least 6 to 8 times to reach your heel

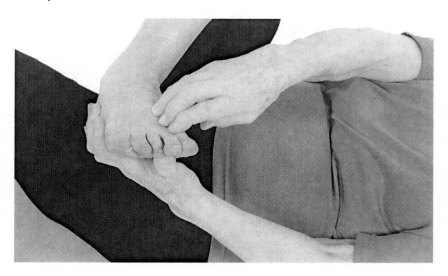

This picture shows how you use your left thumb on the sole of your right foot in self-reflexology and right hand on the top of right foot. The right hand on the top of the right foot moves in the same direction and in the same sequence as the left thumb on the sole of the foot.

I understand that this position may be difficult for many seniors to enable the leg to bend so far as to reach it properly. If you are not flexible enough to reach your foot without stressing the knee, do foot reflexology sitting up.

Use the fingers on the sole of your foot. Refer to the Reflexology Foot chart from time to time so you know what connections you are making with your different organs, glands, and tissues in your body.

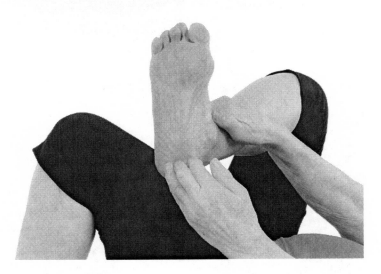

Continue the reflexology on your foot. Remember to hold each reflex point firmly for 10 seconds with deep pressure of approximately 10 to 15 pounds of force all the time. With the right hand, hold right leg above the ankle as shown in the picture.

- Use left fingers together on the heel as your first reflex point; press for 10 seconds

- Move upward step-by-step from the heel until you have covered the entire foot from heel to toes, 7 to 8 steps

- Grasp firmly all your toes together with the left hand; hold for 10 seconds

- Press firmly on the tips of all your toes down with the left hand; hold for 10 seconds. Energy is sent to the brain

- Massage the tip of each toe 10 seconds per toe starting with the baby toe

Self-reflexology is now complete on the right foot. (Use the same procedure on the left foot.) The next and last exercise on the right foot and toes is **yoga**. I chose to demonstrate only one yoga exercise. The description and directions are outlined in the following pages.

YOGA

Why do yoga? Yoga is a gentle, compassionate modality that is able to work with the limits of your body. After an illness, you can help your body recover through the medium of your mind using techniques like yoga, guided visualization, and meditation. Yoga means union of body, mind, and spirit. Yoga is a meditative program that includes exercises to improve flexibility and breathing, decrease stress, and maintain health. In India, yoga has been practiced for centuries as a mental, physical, and spiritual practice based on the principle of mind–body unity. In the western world, yoga is tied into any number of health disciplines and belief systems in a meditation program.

The dictionary meaning of meditation is to engage in a contemplation of reflection. Contemplation means concentration on spiritual things as a form of private devotion. Spirit means the intelligent non-physical part of a person-soul. Soul means the spiritual part of a human being, often regarded as immortal.

Yoga postures are called asanas. Yoga poses force blood out of organs, allowing fresh blood to take its place. This not only cleanses our organs but also provides more nutrients to make our organs stronger and more resistant to disease.

In your human energy system, the center for personal power is located in your solar plexis. This is your third chakra. Your third chakra is linked to your stomach, abdomen, upper GI tract, liver, gallbladder, pancreas, kidney, spleen, adrenal glands, and the middle spine area behind your solar plexus. It is also responsible for the structure of your metabolic system.

Your third chakra handles the energy of your personal power, self-esteem, and personality. Your third chakra is the place where you learn to create boundaries for yourself; issues such as trust, fear of rejection, and self-image are all part of this chakra. This is the center for action, energy, and power.

Stimulation of the solar plexus is an excellent aid to soothe emotional upset. Hara is a line of energy running through the centre of your body. It extends from a few inches under the ribs down toward the pubic bone including the navel. This is the place of power in the body. This means that many nerve centres affecting the balance of the body and mind reside here. It is also the seat of spiritual centres.

Keep the abdominals drawn in—engaged to support the lower back. There are poses to lengthen the hip flexor, to restore the range of motion in the spine, and to stimulate the digestive system. The posture I chose, working specifically on the toes only, will help relax and reduce stress and focus the mind. This posture completes the feet exercises as we stimulate the solar plexus by meditating and contemplating while working on our toes with the fingers. Peace happens when tension leaves your body.

The exercises I demonstrate in my book prove that you and I have such valuable resources available to help us get well and stay well. People may benefit from combining yoga with other exercises and with their conventional medical treatment.

Yoga posture

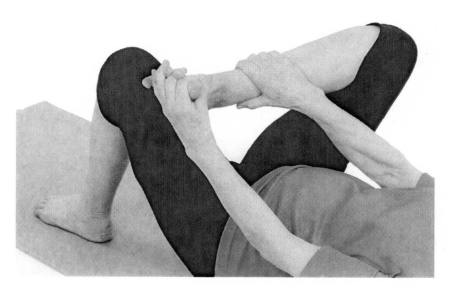

I now will do a yoga exercise on the toes. You will love it! I introduce a multi-purpose idea by moving the toes in several different ways.

- Lay comfortably on your bed
- Interlace your left fingers with your right toes and rotate clockwise for 20 seconds and counterclockwise for 20 seconds
- Move toes up and down for 10 seconds
- Move toes from side to side for 10 seconds
- Do a figure 8 in one direction for 10 seconds
- Do a figure 8 in the opposite direction for 10 seconds
- Rotate toes in one direction for 10 seconds
- Rotate toes in opposite direction for 10 seconds

- Release your fingers and toes and follow the flow of energy, with both hands, from your toes along the leg to the solar plexus

Wasn't that great? Now repeat these reflexology and yoga exercises on your left foot. Follow the same directions as for the right foot.

I believe strongly that this method of energizing your body with self-reflexology and yoga is very effective. If you do self-reflexology it can also save you money. You may feel tuckered out at this point, but don't despair. Rest your body while we do some deep breathing.

DEEP BREATHING

We can live 45 days without food and 7 days without water, but we will die without air in only 2-3 minutes. Our organs, bones, and muscles need to live as well as get extra energy from the air that we breathe; thus, we need to do deep breathing consciously to acquire this benefit. Take deep breaths to fill your lungs fully with life-giving air. As you inhale visualize how oxygen and energy enter the body and reach every cell in the body. Feel the ribcage expand outward, to the side and the back. Shoulders need to stay down and remain relaxed. As you exhale fully, let go and empty the lungs completely of stale air to make room for the next breath. Breathe rhythmically. With each inhale, count 1-4, pause and exhale 5-10 with a slight pause before you inhale again. Do this exercise at least 10 times each day.

This breathing exercise can help the body relax while releasing muscle tightness, worry, fear, and stress. Proper breathing can help us manage chronic pain and overcome physical challenges. This exercise can improve cardiovascular fitness and overall health; it forces you to use your diaphragm muscles. When you take in more air into your lungs, the oxygen replenishes your bloodstream and revitalizes every cell in your body. Think about this wondrous action.

Life-Giving Oxygen Exercise

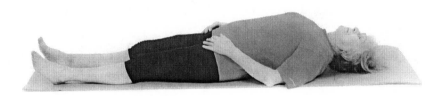

- Lie on your back at ease and rest your hands comfortably on your thighs.
- Inhale through the nose, count 1-4; pause
- Exhale through the mouth, count 5-10, empty lungs completely
- Repeat a minimum of 10 times each day

The millions of cells in your body need life-giving oxygen to function efficiently. Deep breathing is essential to help perform this job. To breathe correctly, you must inhale and then exhale completely in order to squeeze all the impure air from your lungs. Thus the pure oxygen in the bloodstream provides all the muscle cells with vital energy.

FACIAL EXERCISES

When we stimulate and massage facial muscles, we can actually reduce age lines. We can strengthen, tighten, and diminish wrinkles by increasing blood circulation to these muscles. Age lines are reduced; skin and muscles around the brow, mouth, and jaw bone are toned; and the muscles stay firm. Thank God wrinkles don't hurt!

In order to utilize time effectively, I use my feet and legs to enhance the blood and energy circulation in the body and to my face. To do this, I use a tie belt around the bottom of my foot. Please note that the leg is placed in 3 positions during this exercise. These exercises will take time and discipline to master, but I assure you the results are wonderful.

Note: Listen to your body. You may want to omit the leg exercises and simply massage your face and head.

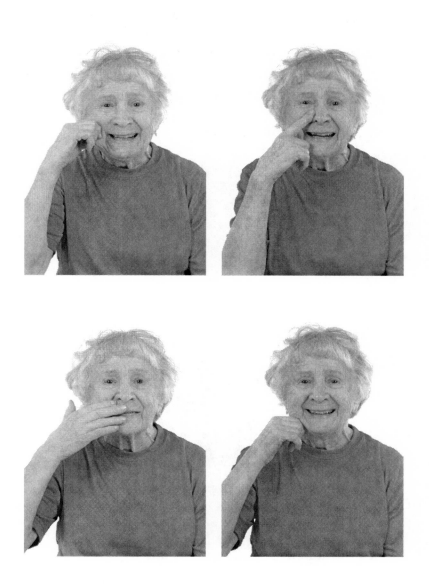

3 Right Leg Positions

1 – Straight up in the air above the body-hamstring stretch

2 – Straight out flat to the right side of the body-inner thigh stretch

3 – Straight up and across the body to the left side (Do not aggravate the hip joint. This position should be avoided if you have a hip replacement.)

Note: May be done with leg bent to 90 degrees, therefore more controlled stretch.

Work Out For The Right Side Of The Face

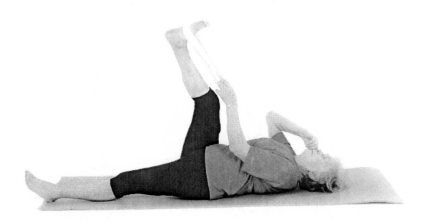

1st right leg position – right leg straight up in the air above the body

- Place belt around the bottom of right foot
- Holding belt in left hand raise right leg straight up in the air above your body

- With the fingers of the right hand, pinch and twist right cheek for 20 seconds
- Massage cheek in one direction for 10 seconds
- Massage cheek in the other direction for 10 seconds
- Together pinch and twist cheek for 10 seconds
- Massage your temple up and down with your fingers and behind your ear with your thumb for 10 seconds
- Manipulate the ear for 5 seconds
- Together pinch and twist cheek for 5 seconds
- Massage cheek for 10 seconds

The massage of the right side of the face takes a total of 90 seconds.

I know this is challenging. Don't give up. You are worth this workout. This exercise may prevent wrinkles if practiced at an early age.

Workout For The Left Side Of The Face

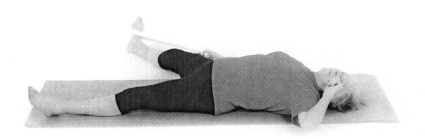

2nd right leg position – flat out to the side of the body

- With your right hand hold belt around the bottom of your right foot as it stretches flat out to the right side of your body
- Repeat the same sequence as described above using your left hand to massage the left side of your face

Workout For The Upper Part Of The Face

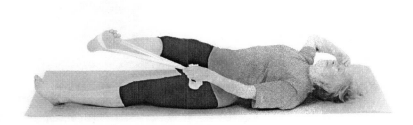

3rd right leg position – straight up and across your body

- With the left hand hold belt around bottom of right foot as you bring your right leg straight across your body; now you will work with the right hand on the upper part of your face
- Massage the middle of your forehead (between your eyebrows) for 10 seconds, moving your hand in a slight slanted angle
- Massage the middle of your forehead (between your eyebrows) in the opposite direction for 10 seconds
- Massage the middle of your forehead (between the eyebrows) up and down for 10 seconds

- Massage right eyebrow for 10 seconds Massage left eyebrow for 10 seconds

- Massage laugh lines along both eyes at the same time for 10 seconds

- Massage forehead from right side to left side and then back again for 10 seconds Massage your nose for 10 seconds

- Massage your forehead, up and down across from right side to left side for 10 seconds

This upper face exercise takes 90 seconds to complete.

Discipline and determination play a large role in doing my exercises. If it's worthwhile to do at all, it's worth doing well. Whoever thinks to massage their ears? We do! They need stimulation too. Realize how much massaging you did in such a short time. Whoever thinks to massage their nose? We do, of course. Our noses will thank us in many ways.

The facial exercises with the 3 right leg positions are now complete.

We will now begin the facial exercises with the 3 left leg positions.

3 Left Leg Positions

1 – Straight up in the air above the body-hamstring stretch

2 – Straight out flat to the left side of the body-inner thigh stretch

3 – Straight up and across the body to the right side (Do not aggravate the hip joint. This position should be avoided if you have a hip replacement.)

Note: May be done with leg bent to 90 degrees, therefore more controlled stretch

Workout For The Right Side Of The Face

1st left leg position – left leg straight up in the air above the body

- Place belt around the bottom of your left foot
- Hold the belt with your left hand
- With your right fingers massage the right sinus area for 10 seconds
- Move to the mouth and massage across your lips from one side to the other for 10 seconds
- Massage the lips up and down for 10 seconds
- Move to the throat and massage your neck with the back of your whole hand across from side to side for 10 seconds (This exercise may prevent the turkey neck.)
- Move to the upper lip and massage up your face along the upper gums towards your right ear for 10 seconds
- Massage and come down along the lower gum line across the side of your face toward the front lower jaw for 10 seconds

You will have massaged for a total of 60 seconds to this point

- With the fingers of your right hand pinch the right side neck muscles under your chin gently pinching from chin to collar bone for 5 seconds; work on the muscles, not just the skin
- Move to the right and pinch muscles upward to the jaw for 5 seconds
- Continue the pattern to the back of your neck counting 5

seconds on each neck area to the count of 85 seconds

- On the last pattern, massage the back of your neck with all fingers for 5 seconds
- This last massage at the back of the neck gives a great relaxing feeling

You have now massaged the right side of your face for a total of 90 seconds. The massage around the mouth area is to get rid of those little river lines and to prevent them from getting deeper and bigger.

I am proud of my wrinkles. They give my face character.

Facial Exercise

2nd left leg position – flat out to the side of the body

Workout for the left side of the face using the same sequence as just described.

- Place the belt around the bottom of left foot
- Hold the belt with the left hand
- With the fingers of your right hand massage the left sinus area for 10 seconds
- Move to the mouth, massaging lips diagonally in one direction for 10 seconds
- Massage lips diagonally in the other direction for 10 seconds
- Move to the throat and massage the neck with the back of your whole hand across from side to side for 10 seconds
- Move to the upper lip and massage up your face along the upper gums towards your left ear for 10 seconds

- Come down along the lower gum line across the side of your face toward the front lower jaw massaging for 10 seconds

You have massaged a total of 60 seconds to this point.

- With the fingers of your right hand pinch the left side neck muscles under your chin gently pinching from chin to collar bone for 5 seconds
- Move to the left and pinch muscles upward to the jaw for 5 seconds
- Continue this pattern to the back of your neck counting 5 seconds on each neck area to the count of 85 seconds
- On the last pattern massage the back of the neck for 5 seconds

You have now massaged the left side of your face for a total of 90 seconds.

There is yet the last massage to benefit your head and hair, as you hold your left leg in the 3rd left leg position—across the body.

Hair needs to be rejuvenated. The cells in the hair follicles need to be stimulated to repair themselves.

Massaging the hair and head with your fingers will encourage this process and make your hair be and look healthy and strong.

Head And Hair Massage

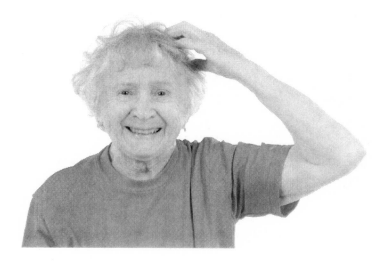

3rd left leg position – left leg across the body

First head/hair exercise

- Place belt at the bottom of your left foot
- Hold belt in right hand. Bring left leg across the body to the right side
- With your left fingers, above the forehead at the hair line, start to massage your scalp upward to the crown of your head to the count of 5 seconds
- Move fingers to the left and massage downward to the hair line for 5 seconds
- Move to the left massage upward to the crown of the head for 5 seconds
- Massage and come down to the hair line for 5 seconds

- Repeat and continue the sequence of up and down massage moving to the left until you have massaged your entire head and come back to the forehead

This head massage will take a total of 60 seconds.

Second head/ hair exercise

- Starting at the front hair line with the fingers of your left hand massage a circle around your head for 10 seconds
- Move upwards and massage another two circles around your head for 10 seconds each

Third head/hair exercise

- The total head exercise count should be 90 seconds. Enjoy the stimulation you have created for your whole head. I am discovering that the colour of my hair is changing and improving. It is not getting lighter and whiter. I can see a hint of strawberry colour. This hair colour is definitely not from a package!

I realize it will take a while to master these instructions. Why use legs with facial exercises? Elevating the feet keeps the legs light with a lot of consistent energy. It is a wonderful way to rest and relax tired feet. It helps the entire body to feel good. And it is a simple way to help prevent and relieve varicose veins. As you move the legs to different positions the back muscles are strengthened and relaxed. This exercise helps and improves balance in your body.

I don't have any difficulty so far doing these exercises. I have yet to have a falling spell in my house.

REFLEXOLOGY & MASSAGE

First, study the reflexology hand chart carefully and follow the directions.

Correctly stimulating reflex points in the hand can induce relaxation and relieve stress and tension in the corresponding glands, organs and tissues in the body. This exercise may slow down the inflammation progression of osteoarthritis in the fingers. As well, it can increase flexibility in the muscles, stimulating blood and energy circulation. Remember there are 4,000 nerve endings in our hands.

Anything worth doing at all is worth doing well.

Energize your body.

Slow down.

Be patient.

Be determined.

Remember: read the chart and directions carefully.

Practice makes perfect. Do it!

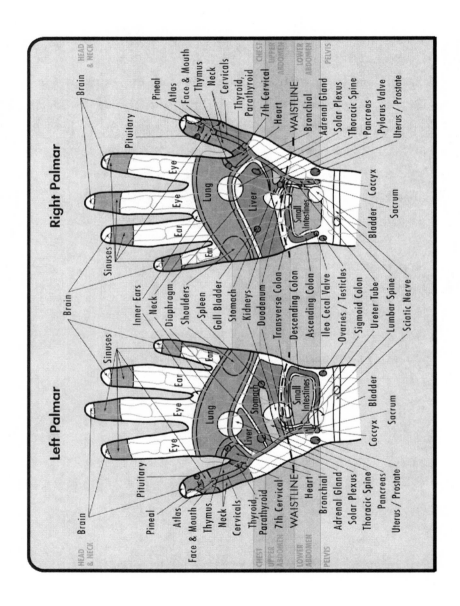

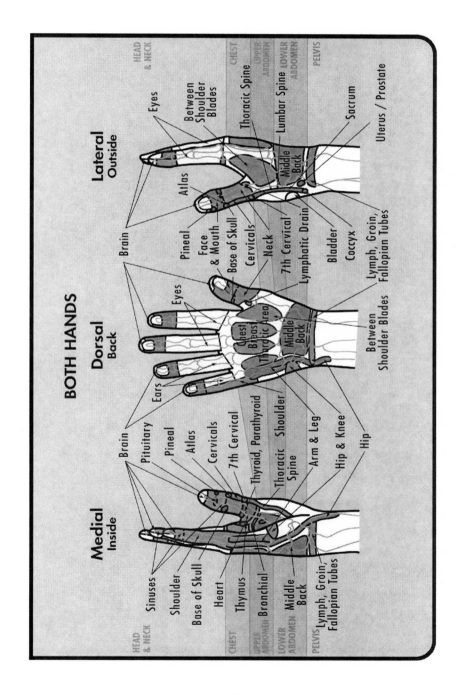

BOTH HANDS

Medial Inside

Dorsal Back

Lateral Outside

HEAD & NECK

CHEST

UPPER ABDOMEN

LOWER ABDOMEN

PELVIS

Sinuses
Shoulder
Base of Skull
Heart
Thymus
Bronchial
Middle Back
Lymph, Groin, Fallopian Tubes

Brain
Pituitary
Pineal
Atlas
Cervicals
7th Cervical
Thyroid, Parathyroid
Thoracic Spine
Arm & Leg
Hip & Knee
Hip

Eyes
Ears
Chest & Breast
Thoracic Area
Middle Back
Between Shoulder Blades

Brain
Eyes
Pineal
Face & Mouth
Base of Skull
Cervicals
Neck
7th Cervical
Lymphatic Drain
Atlas
Bladder
Coccyx
Lymph, Groin, Fallopian Tubes

Eyes
Between Shoulder Blades
Thoracic Spine
Middle Back
Lumbar Spine
Sacrum
Uterus / Prostate

HEAD & NECK
CHEST
UPPER ABDOMEN
LOWER ABDOMEN
PELVIS

Reflexology On Fingers

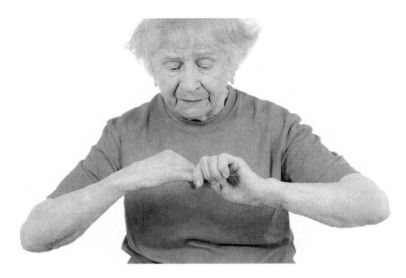

Self-reflexology massage on fingers.

There are 4 parts to the self-reflexology massage on each finger.

There are 2 pull parts, and there are 2 push parts.

The first 2 pull parts are:

- Begin on the right little finger with the left hand
- Grasp the base of the right little finger
- Pull and twist in one direction to the tip count 1
- Grasp the base of the same finger
- Pull and twist in the other direction to the tip count 2
- Do this to the count of 10 on the right little finger

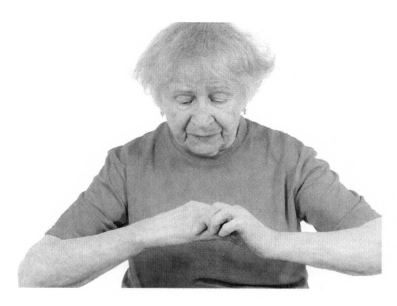

The next 2 parts are 2 push parts of self-reflexology massage on each finger. The energy is being pushed back into the body.

- Grasp at the tip of the right little finger and push to the base of the finger.
- Push and twist in one direction count 1
- Push and twist in the other direction count 2
- Do this to the count of 10 on the right little finger (You have now completed self- reflexology massage on the right little finger)

Next begin to work on your right ring finger. Follow the above directions. Remember to count to 10 with each pull and to the count of 10 with each push.

Again, begin at the base of the finger and follow the same two-step pull-push pattern. Complete the reflexology on every finger and thumb of the right hand. Now, repeat this self-reflexology massage on the fingers and thumb of your left hand using the same two-step pull-push pattern.

This exercise is not as tedious as it sounds. You will be surprised by what you have accomplished so far. Check the reflexology hand chart from time to time. Remember: reflexology means releasing blocked energy in energy pathways of the body. These 12 pathways connect to all of the organs, glands and tissues and culminate in the hands and feet. These pathways should not be blocked if we wish to enjoy vibrant good health.

So far you have worked only on the fingers of both hands. Now you will do reflexology on the right palm with the left thumb.

Reflexology On The Hand

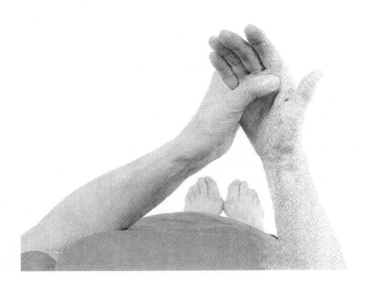

Self-reflexology massage on the right hand

- Begin by manipulating your right fingers somewhat with your left hand

- On the palm of the right hand, just under the base of the forefinger reflex point, apply fine deep pressure of approximately 10 to 15 lbs. of force with your left thumb moving slowly and pulsating firmly down to the wrist and count from 1 to 10

- Feel the pressure

- Then reverse the direction and continue upwards, pulsating along the same path from your wrist to your forefinger and count from 1 to 10

- Note: On the count of 5 your left thumb should be only halfway along your palm

- Place your thumb just under the middle finger reflex point and proceed slowly toward the wrist to the count of 10 and back along the same pathway; count to 10

- Proceed in the same manner under the ring finger and then the baby finger and lastly the thumb; don't forget the thumb; count to 10 in each direction

- While your thumb is pulsating the reflex points on your palm, your left fingers are moving in the same direction stimulating blood circulation on the top of your right hand

This self-reflexology method might seem overwhelming and challenging at first, but you will become more at ease and reap the rewards. Check the hand reflexology chart often. Now follow the same procedure and work across the palm of the right hand.

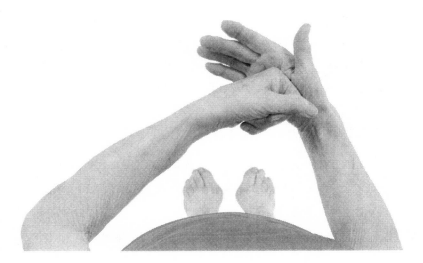

- Next, make a tight fist with your left hand. Run your knuckles firmly, with determination, up and down your whole right palm. Count 1. Repeat this action 10 times

- Next, run your knuckles across your whole right palm. Count 1. Repeat this action 10 times

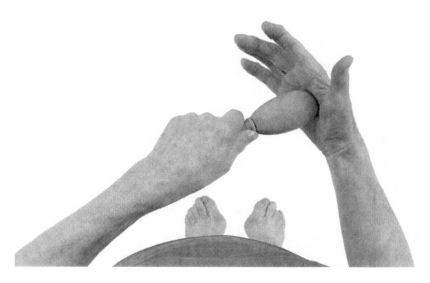

- With left finger tips firmly rotate and massage the right hand palm; count to 10
- With a blunt object, massage the entire palm to the count of 10 (I find a wooden darning tool works well.)
- Press and rub both palms together in one direction and then in the other direction to the count of 10 each way

Hallelujah! Self-massaging the reflexology pressure points in your right hand is now complete. Note: To do reflexology on the palm of the left hand, follow the same procedure as on the right hand.

MASSAGE THE MUSCLES OF YOUR BODY

While doing body massage you become more aware of your own body. Regular body massage increases circulation, and deep massage is one of the most effective non-pharmaceutical treatments for inflammation. Massage can also increase the elasticity of ligaments and muscles, and it has a general relaxing effect on the body. We will start with the forearm, upper arm then move to the torso, finishing with the upper leg and lower leg.

There are three steps to massaging muscles and energizing the rest of your body:

1 – Knead (crush, pinch), with fingers

2 – Twist (clockwise and counter clockwise) with the whole hand

3 – Massage with the whole hand

Note: On the count of 5 you should be halfway on the limb.

Massaging The Arms
Right Forearm Lower Muscles

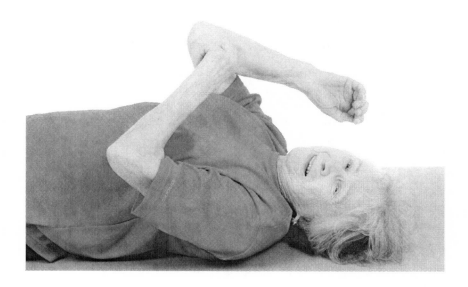

- With the left hand, knead the right lower forearm from wrist to elbow and back to wrist to the count of 10 in each direction; after you finish the lower forearm, repeat this massage on the same right upper forearm; count to 10

- Twist clockwise and counter clockwise starting at the wrist and moving to the elbow to the count of 10 and then back to the wrist to the count of 10

- Massage (rub) from wrist to elbow and back to wrist to the count of 10

Massaging The Arms
Upper Right Arm Muscles

- Massage the muscle of your upper arm in the same three steps as the lower forearm: Knead, twist and massage
- Start at your elbow and work upward to the shoulder
- Knead for 10 seconds upward and back for 10 seconds each on the inner and outer muscles
- Twist for 10 seconds upward and back for 10 seconds each way
- Massage (rub) the whole upper arm for 10 seconds

Massaging your muscles well will help keep them energized. Regular massage can have the effect of reducing painful spasms and areas of muscular tightness. It can strengthen and tone the entire body. As well, it can help to prevent strains and injuries that might otherwise occur, especially when there is already structural damage or weakness. And one of the nicest benefits of massage is the feeling of deep calm. It is thought to be caused by the release of endorphins, which are natural pain killers.

Remember the three parts of massaging muscles and energizing each part of the body:

1 – Knead (crush, pinch)

2 – Twist (clockwise and counter clockwise)

3 – Massage (rub)

Massaging The Torso .

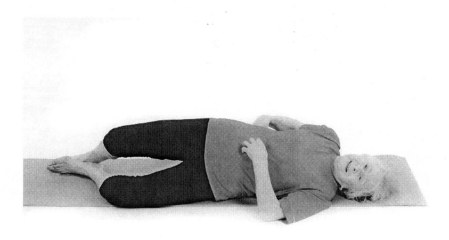

The right side-front and back

Your front and back torso muscles are energized by your fingers.

- Use both hands
- Start at the shoulders with your right hand , reach the right side of the back as best as you can from the shoulders down to the buttocks to the count of 30
- Massage and knead as hard as is comfortable all the way to the groin to the count of 30

These right side torso muscles will thank you as they become energized. The feeling is great! Develop body awareness as you massage various parts of your body. Focus on them and get in touch with them. You will get to know your body, and it is therapeutic.

Massaging The Upper Right Leg

Here is an excellent way to strengthen and energize the thigh muscles in your right leg—the front quadriceps, inside muscle and hamstring.

- With both hands knead the quadriceps from hip to knee to the count of 10 and then knee to hip to the count of 10
- Knead the inside muscle in the same order
- Knead the hamstring in the same order
- With both hands twist each type of muscle in the same order
- Lastly, massage the whole leg to the count of 10

As we age these muscles atrophy, become shorter and weaker. Massaging relaxes and energizes the muscles.

Massaging The Right Lower Leg

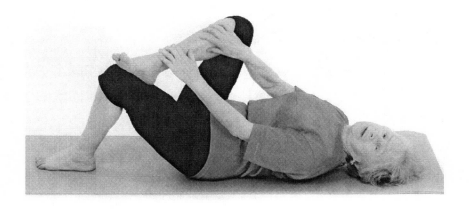

The lower muscles of the right leg also need to be kept strong.

- Knead the front of the right leg and the back of the leg to the count of 10 each way
- Twist the lower leg from knee to ankle and from ankle to knee to the count of 10 each way
- From the knee to the ankle and from the ankle to the knee, massage to the count of 10 each way
- To complete the massage of the right lower leg, return the energy to the solar plexus.
- With both hands together follow the path along the leg and return the energy flowing from your toes to the solar plexus

Congratulations! At this point, you have massaged the entire right side of your body. The left side of your body will now be massaged using the same directions as I have explained for the right side.

Just to remind you, here is the sequence of exercises:

- reflexology on left hand
- massage of left lower arm muscles
- massage left upper arm muscles
- massage torso on left side
- massage left leg from hip to knee
- massage left leg from knee to heel
- complete the massage of the left side of your body by returning the energy to the solar plexus, using both hands following the pathways from your toes, along your leg, torso to solar plexus

When I do my exercise program in the middle of the night, I keep my arms and legs up in the air, working against gravity. The muscles are therefore relaxed. It is a great way to keep arms and legs light with plenty of consistent energy to help the entire body feel well. During a competition in track and field, I experienced running a 200 m sprint that was much easier on my body, and I achieved a much better result—56.46 seconds—because I had elevated my legs for 40 minutes against a wall prior to the race. Try this method and see if it works for you. After a shopping spree or any time your body is fatigued put your feet up at a 45 degree angle. Have a nap. Rejuvenate your wonderful body. I put my feet up when I watch my favorite TV programs, *Wheel of Fortune* and *Jeopardy*. I doze off and miss out on the game show winners. No worries. The winner is my body, mind, and spirit.

SITTING POSITION

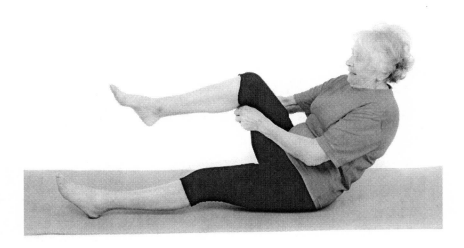

How to sit up from a lying position.

See how easy it is to do.

This method of sitting up from a lying position will eliminate undue stress on your lower back.

- Hold the right leg behind the knee with both hands
- Extend the right leg forward as you bring or swing the body forward to come to a sitting position; you get a more effective abdominal workout without swing

Now you will do some sitting position exercises. Be relaxed as you stretch.

Tune into your body and do not overstretch.

Stretch to prevent and heal muscle soreness and stiffness.

This will get the blood moving and raise your muscle and body temperature. It takes time and sensitivity to stretch properly.

Enjoy. Smile.

Stretch The Upper Hamstrings And Back

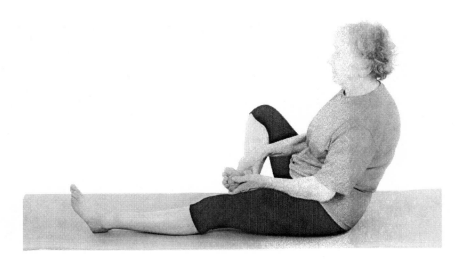

Avoid pulling your foot to overstretch the tendons and ligaments in your ankle.

- Hold onto the outside of your right ankle with left hand
- With your right hand hold above the ankle and press the knee down with your right arm (elbow)
- Gently hold the leg as one unit toward your chest until you feel an easy stretch on the back of your upper leg
- Keep your head forward and hold the stretch for 30 seconds

The upper hamstring and hip muscles will feel an easy stretch.

Stretch For The Back

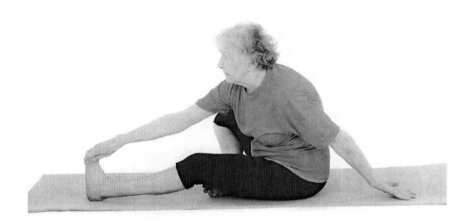

Aim to keep back straight, avoid rounding your back.

- Bend right knee to the floor as you place right foot beside left knee

- With the right hand reach across your body to grasp your left toes or reach as far as is comfortable

- At the same time stretch the left arm behind your body

- Count to 30 seconds as you stretch the muscles in the upper spine, side of lower back as well as hamstrings

Movement should be more from the hip joint not so much as back rounding. This exercise as well will stretch the lower back and between the shoulder blades.

The quadriceps should be soft to the touch. (Relaxed)

Do not dip your head forward. Breathe easily and rhythmically. Change to the left foot and repeat these last 2 sitting exercises.

Stretch The Groin And Hips

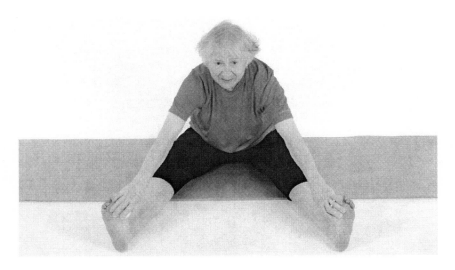

This stretch helps to improve circulation, maintain flexibility and prevent injuries as it loosens up any tight areas in your upper legs and hips. Avoid rounding your upper back and do not reach as far forward. Look straight ahead.

- Sit with feet a comfortable distance apart (90° angle)
- Keep toes and feet relaxed and upright
- With a straight upright back and contracted abdominals slowly lean forward from your hips and try to grasp your toes or as far as is comfortable
- Reach down with your hands and hold your legs at a point that gives an easy stretch for the hamstrings, lower back and hips
- Look ahead and hold the stretch for 30 seconds

Breathe and relax. This exercise is essential in creating balance and stability as you walk.

Stretch The Groin And Hips

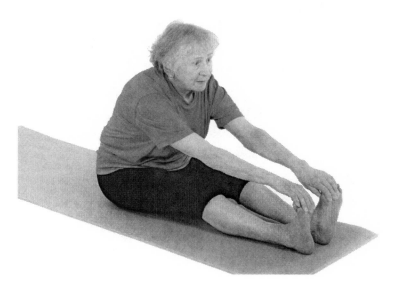

This is a total back muscle stretch exercise. It will increase the stretch in your hamstrings and in your back as far up as the shoulder blades and as far down as the hips.

Avoid rounding your upper back. Reach as far forward as is comfortable. Look straight ahead.

- Stretch both legs together in front of you
- In the same order follow the same directions as you did in the previous exercise
- This exercise requires good overall flexibility
- Hold this stretch for 30 seconds

Sitting Groin Stretch

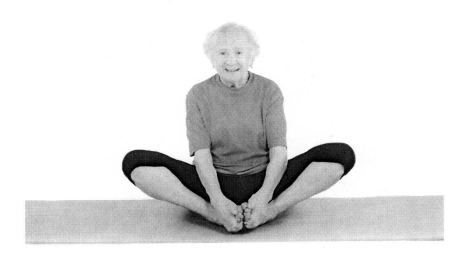

This stretch will limber up your groin area and stabilize tension.

Stretching with control will restore and maintain flexibility and help to develop stability and balance and may prevent cramps in your legs.

- Clasp with your hands the soles of your feet together close to your buttocks

- Gently lean forward from the hips as your elbows press comfortably on the inside of your thighs until you feel an easy stretch in your groin.

- Hold this stretch for 30 seconds

- Relax your jaw and shoulders and breathe rhythmically

- No jerky quick bouncing movements

Enjoy. Be Happy. Smile.

Stretches On The Knees

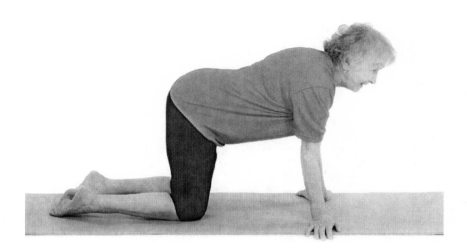

The forearm and wrist stretch

This exercise will improve the flexibility of your hands and wrists.

- Look ahead
- Support yourself on your hands and knees
- Point thumbs to the outside and fingers toward the knees and palms flat
- Lean slightly back to stretch the front, back and inside parts of your forearms, fingers and wrists
- Hold for 30 seconds

You may find you are very tight in this area. Relax and stretch again.

Stretch For The Back, Shoulders, Arms And Fingers

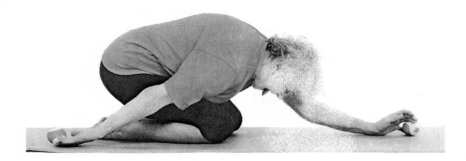

This exercise can reduce tension and increase flexibility in the shoulders, arms, fingers, sides, upper and lower back. Use the sponge balls.

- From a kneeling position, sit comfortably on your heels and your forehead almost on the floor
- With a sponge ball in each hand, extend far and stretch arms in opposite directions, squeeze balls for 30 seconds
- Change arms direction and stretch and again squeeze sponge balls for 30 seconds

At the same time you do this exercise, why not give your tongue a workout. Stretch it out as far as you can and let it hang loose. Pout your cheeks, stretch your lips, open your nostrils.

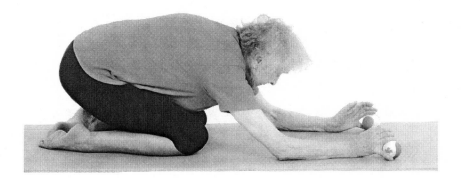

Sponge balls strengthen the muscles in your hands and wrists and increase flexibility in the muscles stimulating blood and energy circulation.

- From a kneeling position, sit comfortably on your heels and forehead almost on the floor
- Bring both arms forward and squeeze balls between each finger as previously described at the beginning of this chapter
- Squeeze balls between baby and ring fingers to the count of 10
- Balls between ring finger and middle finger to the count of 10
- Balls between middle finger and forefinger to the count of 10
- Balls between forefinger and thumb to the count of 10

Nobody else notices my funny face when I do this humorous exercise! All the muscles of your body need to be stretched and exercised.

Remember that so far you have exercised your ears, your nose, and now your tongue, etc. I believe this is quite an accomplishment, don't you?

FORWARD SPLITS

At this point, your body has been warmed up with all the stretching, massaging, reflexology and yoga.

This forward splits exercise, I believe, helps the balance in my body and flexibility in my legs so that I am still able at the age of 95 to make long strides as I walk with a relatively good posture. No baby or chicken steps for me! Doing this exercise will help you enjoy walking. Head over shoulders, shoulders over hips. Look ahead and smile.

Learning to do the splits takes time and regular practice. It may be somewhat challenging for you at first, but don't despair. Let your body gradually adapt to the physical changes needed to accomplish the splits comfortably. I am not trying to discourage you from trying to do the forward splits.

Be certain not to overstretch. Do not rush and injure yourself. Don't fret if you are unable to do the splits. Use control as you find the proper stretch feeling. Don't get paranoid reading this. Be brave. If I can do it, so can you! Just try. For everyday living, being able to do the splits is hardly necessary.

Be brave, and be different.

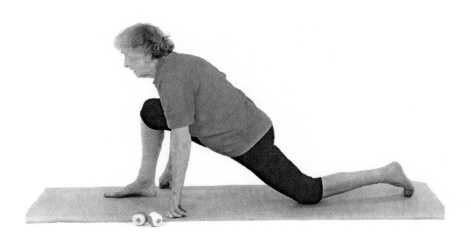

All the lower muscles from the hips will be stretched.

This controlled hip flexor stretch stretches the front of the hips, groin, shin of the back leg, and the buttocks of the front leg.

If the toes on back leg are curled under, you might get a calf stretch.

- Look straight ahead
- In a kneeling position move one leg forward until the knee of the forward leg is directly over the ankle
- Your other knee should be resting on the mat
- Lower the front of your hips downward to create an easy stretch
- Hold 10–20 counts (I hold 30 counts. You too will be able to, after practice.)

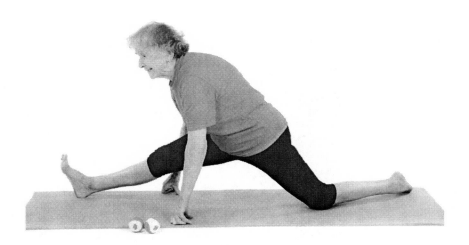

- Move the foot forward until you feel a controlled easy stretch in the back of your leg and groin; hold 5–15 seconds; relax
- Now slowly stretch the foot a little farther, a fraction of an inch each time until you again feel a mild tension; hold 5–10 seconds; relax
- Extend straight the whole leg as far as you can; hold 30 seconds; relax; flex and point toes 15 seconds each
- Lower your hips straight down; shoulders should be over the hips
- Increase these stretches gradually; stretch the other leg
- Be in control; use your hands for balance and stability (If the stretch tension increases as you stretch or it becomes painful, you are stretching too far. Relax.)

The hamstrings, quadriceps, and especially the calf muscles will be energized and strengthened. Good posture and balance will be hugely improved as you walk. Be certain to work both exercises on each leg.

This is the end of the stretching exercises from *The O.K. Way to a Healthy, Happy Life*. These stretching exercises are my favorite cure for insomnia. Several times a week, in the middle of the night, after completing these exercises, I will get a drink of water, visit the bathroom, and put on my bed socks. I love to plump up my feather pillow and snuggle under my down quilt, and soon I am in slumber land until nine or ten a.m.

Stretching is peaceful, relaxing, and definitely not competitive. Exercising helps keep muscles supple and flexible, and prevents common injuries. Anybody and everyone needs to stretch to relax the mind and tune up the body. Regular stretching will help you develop body awareness of the various parts of your body. You get to know yourself. Body, mind and spirit are in harmony constantly.

For further motivation, exercise with a friend or friends on a regular basis. But don't compare yourself with others. Proper stretching means stretching within your own limits, being relaxed, and avoiding comparisons with what other people can do.

"If exercise could be packed into a pill,
it would be the single most prescribed and beneficial
medication in the nation."
— *Robert Butler, MD BC Health Guide Healthwise*

Your homework assignment:

Treat your body as your friend, not a stranger. Be sensitive towards it. Watch it. Listen to it.

Love your body. Observe its needs and its requests and even have fun. Be sensitive to being alive. Do the exercises I have described in this chapter to the best of your ability. I know you will benefit greatly from the effort. If you have any medical conditions, please check with your doctor before beginning any exercise program.

After an illness, you can help your body recover through the medium of your mind when you use techniques like yoga, guided visualization, and meditation.

Exercise is the best medicine. The body is strengthened; the mind is alert; the spirit is free.

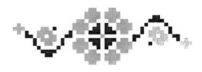

A middle-aged woman has a heart attack and is taken to the hospital. While on the operating table she has a near death experience. During that experience she sees God and asks him if this is the end for her. God says: "No." He explains that she has another 30 years to live.

Upon recovery, she decides to stay in the hospital and have a face lift, liposuction, breast augmentation, and a tummy tuck. She even has someone come in and change her hair colour and give her a new hairstyle. She figures if she's got another 30 years to live she might as well make the most of it.

She walks out of the hospital after the last operation and is killed by an ambulance speeding up to the emergency entrance.

She arrives before God and complains: "I thought you said I had another 30 years!"

God replies, "I didn't recognize you."

Eight
Nutrition & Recipes

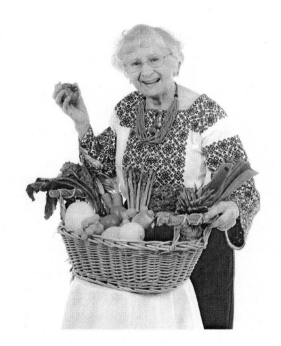

Fresh fruits and vegetables are vital for vibrant
good health. That includes tomatoes!

Lesson: Good food is the first line of defense for achieving and maintaining a healthy, vibrant body. If you eat the right foods, you can add years to your life and offset the signs of premature aging. By making healthy choices you will enjoy a more active, healthy, and independent life. Nourish your body with healthful foods in moderate amounts, and they will provide the fuel to function during the day.

"The power of food and positive thinking may change your life."
— *Adam Hart*

One of the questions I am asked most frequently is: "Olga, what do you eat?" I will tell you: "Everything." I was blessed with a strong constitution. I digest my food well, and I am not allergic to anything that I know of. I try to eat healthily most of the time, and I believe that if I am good 80% of the time, my body can take care of the other 20%.

One of the pleasures of daily exercise is the ability to eat more because you burn so many calories. I love nothing better than a good steak, baked potato, lots of brightly coloured vegetables, and a glass of red wine. I crave things like raw fruit, broccoli, and carrots. I love Italian food, and I do have a sweet tooth, but I try to be sensible. I don't overeat, and I only eat when I'm hungry. I eat good, wholesome food in moderate amounts, and I enjoy 4 to 5 small meals a day. I believe if a person wants to be healthy and have lifelong vitality, he/she should not overeat but try to eat food that packs the greatest nutritional benefits—food that is fresh, natural, unprocessed, and unrefined. I believe in the saying, "You are what you eat."

I like breakfast. A good morning meal brightens any day, and it sets the tone and mood for the rest of the day, be it a bowl of hot cereal or an egg and buttered toast with homemade jam.

Breakfast is an important meal. Eat a good breakfast, and you start the day off on the right track. You want to plan an enjoyable afternoon 'second lunch' that helps to energize the end of your work day and curb your appetite for dinner when you will eat a little bit less.

Here is an example of typical meals I would eat in one day.

Breakfast:

Juice

Hot cereal (Oatmeal or Red River cereal on alternate days) with a handful of grapes

Milk 2 %

Grapes - a handful fresh green or red

Coffee - ½ tsp instant coffee mixed with 1 tsp Krakus (100% caffeine free instant coffee substitute, a product of Poland made of roasted barley, chicory, rye, beet roots)

Brown toast

Peanut butter, honey or jam (My homemade blueberry, black-berry or strawberry jams.)

Egg - soft boiled or fried sunny-side up

Mid-morning snack:

Whole wheat bagel & cheese

Raw carrot

Nuts - handful

Tropicana orange juice (lots of pulp)

Lunch

Soup, homemade (Chicken noodle, broccoli, pea, vegetable)

Sandwich (Salmon or tuna, egg or roast beef; no pre-packaged or deli meats)

Salad, fruit or vegetable, raw and fresh

Milk

Mid-afternoon snack

Nuts – handful

Tossed green salad

Yogurt

Tropicana orange juice or tea

Supper:

Chicken (roasted drumstick with Thai sweet chili sauce)

Rice

Sautéed vegetables (onion, garlic, green peppers, tomatoes)

Raspberries with yogurt

I look forward to a glass of red wine with dinner or while watching *The Wheel of Fortune* and *Jeopardy* with my legs propped at a 45° angle.

Eating 4 to 5 smaller meals each day is a good habit to develop. Eating slowly lets the brain know that you have eaten enough. The best time to eat a larger meal is early in the day, especially in the summertime. It encourages a healthy metabolism and discourages both weight gain and mid-day sluggishness. Follow these daily goals: wake up ready for breakfast, get your fuel by day, and diet or fast by night. Did you know you lose unwanted body fat when you are sleeping?

My grocery list consists primarily of fresh B.C. products. I also benefit from the many vegetables that I grow in my garden. In summer, the fresh produce is so bountiful it provides enough fuel to generate energy for the rest of the day. Good quality chocolate is advisable in small amounts. Researchers have found that it can reduce the risk of cardiovascular disease by 37 per cent and stroke by 29 per cent. Any way you want to measure it, chocolate in moderation is good for you. I like a daily glass of red wine or an occasional glass of scotch, for its medicinal properties.

Here is a list of other healthy foods I make part of my nutrition plan.

Garlic: I eat it regularly. It boosts your immune system, has very real effects on bacteria, viruses, yeast, and parasites. It breaks down the plaque in the cardiovascular system that builds up in the arteries, gets rid of tumours, and prevents stroke and heart attack. Prevention is the best strategy for a strong and healthy cardiovascular system.

Wild salmon: This omega 3 fatty acid-rich, lean fish is full of protein and vitamins D, B–12, niacin, selenium, and magnesium. It reduces inflammation, risk of blood clots, and slows down the progress of cognitive disease such as Alzheimer's.

Nuts: Almonds, walnuts, hazelnuts, and chestnuts are high in fibre that helps lower cholesterol. They are rich in omega 3 fatty acids that can prevent heart disease and contain plant nutrients with vitamin E and selenium that act as antioxidants.

Blueberries: Nature's candy. Sweetness with a punch. This lovely fruit is rich in antioxidants that help slow down the aging process and protect us against disease. Try blueberries sprinkled over your cereal or yogurt, or throw them into the blender with grapes to produce a powerful antioxidant juice or smoothie.

Beets: They are a great source of iron and the pigment, betalains, helps to support liver detoxification. Borsch is like medicine.

Swiss Chard: This leafy green vegetable is high in phytonutrients, which are powerful anti- inflammatory agents. Chard is a natural energy booster.

Ginger: This energizing herb not only reduces inflammation, but it alleviates bloating while calming digestive upsets.

Pineapple: Bromelain, the enzyme found in this tropical fruit, improves digestion by helping absorb proteins. It contains manganese needed for bone development

Tahini: My mother may never have tasted tahini, but I have come to love the rich, creamy paste made from hulled, toasted sesame seeds. It adds a mild nutty flavor to sauces, dips and dressings. Tahini is loaded with B vitamins for our brain and nervous system, and fatty acids that give us glowing, healthy skin. The vitamin E and other antioxidants in tahini help slow down the aging process. The calcium in sesame seeds is more digestible and absorbable than calcium from cow's milk or other dairy sources.

Quinoa: Is it a grain, bean, or a nut? Pronounced "Qin-Wah", this grain-like superfood is grown for its edible seeds. It originates from South and Central America and Peru. Quinoa was once considered a sacred food by the Incas who called it "Mother of all Grains". It cooks up light and fluffy and goes well with both sweet and savoury foods. It is full of essential amino acids, fibre, and calcium and is gluten-free. My mother never tasted quinoa, but I find it one of the healthiest foods I enjoy.

My family, like many others at the time, was built on rock-solid, dependable and hard-working prairie stock. Although we never went hungry, even during the worst of the Great Depression, we all worked hard to put food on the table. We grew all our vegetables, raised our own animals, foraged for indigenous foods, and picked wild berries and mushrooms. You have never tasted a real strawberry unless you have tasted a ripe, wild strawberry still warm from the sun.

We picked gooseberries, the first berry to appear in the prairie spring. I would take a little bucket and pick them on my way back from school. We also picked blueberries, currants and, of course, Saskatoon berries that were quite plentiful. My brothers, sisters, and I picked, on average, five pails of Saskatoon berries, so mother could fill quart jars with delicious Saskatoon berry preserves for the cold winters.

Other wild foods we enjoyed were mushrooms. We were able to identify five or six different edible wild mushrooms. Of course, it was important to know which ones were and were not poisonous. Yet there was even a use for the lethal mushrooms. We would bring the poisonous ones home, and mother would put them in sugar and water, and this natural pesticide effectively killed house flies. Different mushrooms grew at different times. One of my favorites is the tall, black morels. Mother would make delicious sauces and soups with these wild mushrooms, and she would dry them to preserve them to use through the year. If I close my eyes, I can still taste her delicious mushroom soup.

As for domestic foods, we had dairy cows, beef, and we always had pork, chickens, turkeys, geese, and ducks. We had a smoker and cured our own hams and made our own sausage. Our dairy cows provided good, wholesome milk that we transformed into butter, cream, cheese, or yogurt. Eventually, mother learned how to make solid cheese by adding rennet to the milk.

We had two or three humungous gardens, and all of the children had to help with the weeding. Everything was grown organically. There were no poisonous herbicides and pesticides. Since we were able to grow most of our foods, there were only a few things we needed to buy, such as apples, oranges, and tomatoes. I was about 12 years old when I tasted my first tomato.

We had an ice house located in the basement of the summer kitchen, a separate building from the main house where the kitchen was only occupied in the summer, where three meals were prepared each day. In winter, men would cut large chunks of ice from the frozen pond and haul it up to the summer kitchen basement and cover the ice in layers with sawdust. These blocks of ice would remain frozen until the next winter. This was our refrigerator.

Since Dad was a wheat farmer, we always had enough grain to sell and to keep for our personal use. He would take the wheat to be milled at the flour mill, and we had all the wheat flour we needed. Mother made all our bread and homemade noodles. You can just imagine how much bread you need to bake for up to 15 people. She baked twice a week, keeping the starter dough warm under a blanket at night. She would start making bread in the morning and put these huge loaves in roasters to rise. She baked the loaves in the outdoor oven, called a *pich*. The fragrance coming from those baking loaves was home-made medicine.

An excellent way to get good wholesome food organically grown in fertile soil is to plant and tend a garden. Now I spend many happy hours working in my vegetable garden with the birds and the bees for company, and I benefit from the fresh air, exercise and, of course, the harvest.

Gardening is increasingly becoming a popular hobby as people realize the benefits for body, mind, and soul, not to mention their pocketbooks if they can grow their own fruits and vegetables.

As some people age, they may start to ignore the quality and quantity of their food. As the need for calories decreases, the need for nutrients often increases. As we age, we need so little, but that little can mean so much. Remember, you cannot stay healthy by eating only tea and toast for breakfast, lunch, and supper, or by munching a tomato over the sink because you don't want to dirty your dishes! Food is fuel. It doesn't have to be a big meal. We're holding onto the old idea of someone slaving away in the kitchen preparing meals for the family. We all enjoy planning meals and cooking for two or more, but even if you are single take the time to eat properly. Your food is the first line of defense for achieving and maintaining a healthy vibrant body. Healthy choices enable you to enjoy a more active and independent life.

Plan your meals in advance, and choose your food wisely and intelligently: pick foods rich in vitamins, minerals, and nutrients. We have one body and one mind for life. It's our responsibility to take care of them.

"Use it or lose it."

As I was collecting some of my favorite recipes to include in the book, I came across *The Blue Ribbon Cookbook*, a well-worn little book that dates back to 1905. As a child, I remember seeing it in my mother's kitchen. The section called "Healthy Eating for Seniors" is quite interesting and, despite being written over one hundred years ago, the advice is logical and still useful, so I will include it.

The diet of the aged should suit their individual condition. If fat, heavy and sleepy, inclined to sit and slumber, let them avoid fat meats, butter, sugar and fat-creating elements of food: and, instead, eat lean meat, brown bread, fish, nuts, vegetables and fruits, with the usual quantities of tea or coffee. Buttermilk is one of the most desirable foods for old people, as it prevents the transformation of the cartilaginous tissue, which enters into the formation of tendons, arteries, etc, - into bone, thus largely relieving the stiffness to which old age is liable, as well as ameliorating its infirmities in other ways.

On the contrary, if they are lean, querulous of sleepless, let them eat of fat meat, bread and butter, buckwheat cakes, rice, milk, buttermilk, potatoes, etc., and the better nourishment of the system will manifest itself in improved sleep and disposition.

A healthy diet provides the ingredients to build and repair bones and tissues and keeps the complex workings of the human body functioning optimally. It also provides the mental and physical energy necessary for your daily life - work, recreation, relationships and time with family. It is clear that a healthy diet also protects us from infectious illnesses and chronic diseases, so that we may age with a minimum of ill health, pain and disability.

A healthy diet should consist of 25% meat, dairy products, beans, and grains while 75% of a healthy diet should consist of brightly coloured fruits and vegetables, fermented foods, such as buttermilk, yogurt, sauerkraut and, of course, herbs and spices.

Today, there is a growing movement to try to eat locally grown food as much as possible. Eating seasonal food is good for your health and for the environment. I think that if you live in a tropical climate, where fresh vegetable and fruits are available all year round, it might be possible to live only on raw food. I enjoy eating raw vegetables and fruits in season but, personally, I find when living in a colder northern country like Canada that I need a certain amount of cooked food.

It is wonderful that more and more people are becoming interested in making healthy fermented foods, such as sauerkraut, yogurt, and pickles. Oh, the wonderful power of sauerkraut! The healthful quality of sauerkraut was recognized as far back as 200 BC, when history records it was served to the laborers working on the Great Wall of China.

Good health begins with good nutrition; naturally fermented foods are healthy, safe, and fairly easy to produce. If it were not safe, I wouldn't be here! My parents would make huge vats of pickles and sauerkraut. The important thing to remember when making fermented foods is to make sure the vegetables are submerged under liquid. This prevents them from molding.

In this age of processed and synthetic foods, whole foods like sauerkraut are more important than ever. Fermented foods, such as sauerkraut, sourdough bread, miso, tempeh, tamari, chutney, yogurt, cultured butter and cheese are products in lactic-acid fermented foods. Fermentation neutralizes unhealthy chemicals in raw foods and adds a host of beneficial microorganisms to foods. The fermentation makes the food more digestible and increases the healthy flora in our intestinal tracts. Sauerkraut, a powerhouse of superior lactic acid, enzymes, and other important nutrients improves health and even cures many common ailments. To retain its full flavour, serve it raw or barely heated through. Cooking makes kraut milder. Sauerkraut juice is a nutritious drink, but it's powerful: two swallows is usually enough for me.

The natural properties of sauerkraut, and its juices, strengthen the acidity of the stomach, prevent constipation, encourage function of the pancreas, and stimulate the secretions of all digestive juices. It cleanses the blood and neutralizes unhealthy chemicals found in many foods. Also, it supports natural resistance against infections and strengthens the body's immune system.

This following is a small sample of my favorite recipes—mainly traditional. The recipe for homemade sauerkraut is easy to make. How long you ferment it depends on your preference and personal taste. Taste your sauerkraut to determine when it reaches the state you prefer. It will get stronger and less firm as it ages. Move it to the fridge to slow the process. Try it. Eat healthy. *Bon Appetite*!

Sauerkraut #1

Shred cabbage very finely and pack in a quart jar.

With the handle of a wooden spoon, make a hole in the cabbage to the bottom of the jar. Add 1 teaspoon of pickling salt.

Fill the jar with boiling water and seal.

Keep the jar in a cool, dark place, and the sauerkraut will be ready to enjoy in a week.

Sauerkraut # 2

1 1/2 lb cabbage finely shredded

2 1/2 tsp coarse salt

1 carrot shredded (optional)

1 medium onion, thinly sliced

1 tsp pickling spices

Mix all the vegetables and spices together. Sprinkle with salt and mix thoroughly.

Pack firmly into a crock or jar and let the brine (kraut juice) come over top of the cabbage. Put a plate on top of the cabbage. Fill a quart jar with water and seal. Place this jar as a weight on the plate. Cover and let stay in a medium warm place for the vegetables to ferment—1–3 weeks.

When the fermentation has ceased, fill the sauerkraut into sealers, seal tightly, and store in a cool place (in the fridge). Kraut also stores well by freezing in containers and freezer bags.

Sauerkraut Soup (Kapusnyak)

1 lb fresh spare ribs or smoked pork shank

6-8 cups water as needed

1 medium onion chopped

1 cup sauerkraut, drained (save the juice)

Salt and pepper

Chopped dill or parsley

1 cup chopped mushrooms, canned or fresh (optional)

1 medium potato, diced

1 medium carrot, sliced

2 tablespoons flour

1–2 tablespoons butter

Wash the ribs and cut them apart. In the pot that is used for cooking the soup, brown the ribs first. Then add the onions to fry. Cover with water and simmer for about an hour. May add more water if needed. Squeeze the sauerkraut, but save the juice. Add sauerkraut, potato and carrot and continue simmering until vegetables are tender—about 30 minutes. Brown the flour lightly in the butter. Add some soup liquid into it and stir until smooth and return it to the soup and to a boil.

Season to taste and flavor with dill or parsley.

Serve the meat as a separate course or place a small piece of it into each bowl of soup, which is usually served with rye bread. Serves: 6–8.

The following recipes are some of my personal favorites. Some of them are truly healthy and can be eaten daily. Some of these exceptional recipes are my guilty pleasures and they are not to be eaten daily, but when I do cook them, I thoroughly enjoy them.

Bon Appetite! As Ukrainians say *Smachnoho!*

Buckwheat Casserole

1 cup buckwheat

3 cups boiling water

1 medium onion chopped

3 tbsp. butter

½ lb garlic sausage or any other sausage

1 tsp. salt

1 tsp. sugar

Preheat oven to 350 °

Cook buckwheat in boiling water until all the water is absorbed.

In the meantime, put 3 tbsp butter in a frying pan. Add the chopped onion and peeled, sliced garlic sausage. Fry together until the onion is well sautéed. Pour over the buckwheat. Add salt and sugar. Mix well and place into a small greased casserole dish. Bake at 350° for ¾ of an hour.

May be served with an entrée course or enjoyed as a luncheon dish.

Borsch

1 lb fresh spare ribs (optional)

8 cups water

1 teaspoon salt

large onion chopped

2 cups chopped cabbage

1 can tomato soup

2 cups diced canned tomatoes

1 can beans

2 large beets, cut in very thin strips, also use tops (leaves, chopped)

1 large carrot, sliced thin

1 cup potatoes diced

1 clove garlic, finely diced

Chopped dill

Salt and pepper

Sour cream

Wash the ribs and cut them apart. In the pot in which the soup will be cooking, first brown the ribs. Add and fry the onions and garlic. Cover with water, bring to a boil, and simmer for about 1½–2 hours. Skim the foamy substance that comes to the top during boiling. You may add more water as needed. Add the beets, carrots, cabbage, and simmer until meat and vegetables are tender—about 3/4 hour. Add tomato soup, tomatoes, and beans. Bring to a boil and simmer another ½ hour.

One tablespoon of sour cream is placed in each bowl of borsch. It tastes better when the cream is added just before serving. Enjoy!! It's a meal in itself. Serves 6–8 people. (I believe in bountiful batches.)

Boastfully, Ukrainians claim their borsch as the only genuine borsch in the world, being the national soup of Ukraine.

Broccoli Soup

2–3 broccoli bunches cut up

2 tablespoons butter

1 medium onion, chopped

1–2 carrots sliced

Salt and pepper

Fry the onion in butter till golden color. Add broccoli and carrots and sauté. Cover the vegetables with enough water to just cover and cook for ½ hour until vegetables are tender. Season with salt and pepper. Cool. Puree the vegetables. Portion soup into containers and freeze. Label.

To enjoy the soup, thaw it out of the freezer. To 4 tablespoons heaping vegetables, add chicken or beef stock or milk. Season for flavour. Bring to a boil.

Enjoy with soda crackers. Use your imagination as to the quantity of vegetables you need to use. You may wish to double the recipe.

I use this same method to make other soups, like carrot soup, pea soup, or potato soup. Create your own recipes. That's how new recipes are made.

Cornmeal Casserole
Nachynka Bukovinian Style

5 tbsp butter

1 onion chopped fine

1 tsp sugar

1 tsp salt

¼ tsp pepper

1 cup cornmeal

3 ½ cups scalded milk

½ cup light cream

3 eggs beaten well

Sauté onion in butter until tender. Add the cornmeal, salt, sugar and pepper to butter onion mixture. Mix thoroughly so that the cornmeal would be well coated with butter. Pour in the scalded milk gradually, stirring briskly until mixture is smooth. Cook on medium heat stirring constantly until thickened. Remove from heat and blend in the cream, then fold in well-beaten eggs. Spoon into a 2-quart buttered casserole dish.

Bake the *nachynka* uncovered in a moderate oven at 350 degrees for 1 hour. Well baked *nachynka* should have a crisp golden crust on top and sides. Serves 6-8.

Serve this like Yorkshire pudding with a meat course or as a luncheon dish with sour cream and cottage cheese.

Onion Salad

6 sweet onions, finely sliced

1 ½ cups water

1 ½ cups white vinegar

2 cups sugar

3 tsp salt

½ cups mayonnaise

3 tsp celery seeds

salt and pepper to taste

To make brine, heat water, vinegar, sugar, and salt to boiling. Pour over onions. After 3 - 5 hours drain brine from the onions. Combine mayonnaise, celery seeds, salt, and pepper and add to onions. Onions in the brine can keep in the fridge for a month.

Carrot Salad

2 lbs carrots, sliced

2 sweet onions, sliced

1 green pepper, sliced

1 15oz can tomato soup

1 cup sugar

1 tsp salt

1/ tsp pepper

½ cup salad oil

¼ cup white vinegar

Cook carrots until tender but crisp. Combine onions and pepper. Combine remaining ingredients for the sauce and bring to a boil. Pour hot brine over carrots, onions and pepper. Chill and store in the fridge.

3 Bean Salad

1 19oz can chickpeas, drained

1 14oz can green beans, drained

1 14oz can yellow wax beans, drained

1 14oz can kidney beans, rinsed

½ cup green pepper, chopped

½ cup onions, chopped

½ cup salad oil

½ cup vinegar

½ cup sugar

Mix well the last three ingredients until sugar is completely dissolved. Combine all ingredients and refrigerate at least one day for best flavour.

Tapioca Pudding

This is an oldie but goodie. I just love it!

½ cup tapioca

4 eggs

½ cup sugar

½ cup raisins, rinsed

2 tbsp melted butter

1 qt milk

¼ tsp salt

1 tsp Blue Ribbon vanilla

cinnamon

Soak tapioca in milk overnight. Beat the eggs and sugar together until light. Add the salt, vanilla, raisins, cinnamon, and butter. Bake in a casserole in a moderate over 350°F for one hour. Serve hot or cold with medium cream.

Pyrogies

Without a doubt, pyrogies are the ultimate Ukrainian comfort food! Now that you can find pyrogies in the freezer section of most grocery stores anyone can enjoy our national culinary treasure any time they want. Nothing beats homemade.

The recipe below will make about 6 dozen.

Dough:

5-6 cups all-purpose flour

¾ cup each water and milk, warmed

3-5 tbsp melted butter or oil

2 eggs

1 tsp salt

Variation: For the pyrogie dough replace water and milk with 3-4 tbsp mashed potatoes and 1 ½ cups potato water.

Dough: Combine water, milk, butter, and eggs, beating well. Stir in flour and salt. Knead dough on floured surface about two minutes, until smooth and soft. Place in a lightly oiled bowl, cover, and let rest at least 30 minutes.

Potato Filling:

1 onion finely chopped

¼ cup butter

3 cups mashed potatoes

1 cup cheddar cheese grated

Salt and pepper to taste

Prepare the filling by frying the onion in butter. Combine onion, potato, and cheese. Season to taste. Cool.

Work with half of the dough at a time. Roll out on a floured surface until approximately 1/8" thick. Cut circles of dough using a round cookie cutter or cut 2 ½ inch squares with a knife.

Place a rounded teaspoon of filling in the centre of each circle. Fold over and form a half circle, and use your fingers to pinch the edges firmly together to seal in the filling. Squares will form triangles when pinched. This recipe should make more than 5 dozen pyrogies. Place on a very clean tea towel and cover to prevent drying.

Bring a large pot of water to boil and, when boiling, gently place about 10 pyrogies one at a time into the water. Boil for 6-7 minutes. Stir them around to prevent sticking. When they cook, they will float to the top.

Remove carefully with a slotted spoon and transfer to a casserole dish. Add butter or oil and toss gently to coat the pyrogies with the butter so they do not stick.

There are several variations you can try. Mix potato filling with sautéed mushrooms, with sautéed sauerkraut, or with dry curd cottage cheese.

Use any kind of dried fruit or fresh berries like prunes, blueberries, or Saskatoon berries with a little bit of sugar. Soak prunes for 2 hours in warm water. Cook the prunes and mash them for the filling. Not too mushy.

On the dough circle/square put just enough filling so that it will seal well. With experience, you will find the filling leaks out because it had too much juice or was not pinched carefully enough to seal well.

Cream sauce for pyrogies

1 onion, medium, chopped
3 tbsp butter
1 lb fresh mushrooms, chopped
1 can cream of mushroom soup

Fry the onion until transparent. Add and sautée mushrooms. Dilute the soup with a little bit of milk and stir into the onion and mushroom mixture. Simmer for 10-15 minutes. I have had rave reviews about this sauce.

I serve pyrogies with sour cream, but some people also add crisp, crumbled bacon and fried onions.

Pyrogies may be cooked and then pan-fried in butter until golden brown.

Raw pyrogies may be arranged on trays, covered with a tea towel and frozen, and then placed in freezer bags to freezer. When you are hungry and ready to enjoy eating pyrogies, boil them as instructed above. This method will take longer because the boiling water will cool off until it starts to boil again.

Be patient. Be careful. Have lots of fried onions ready. Have a healthy appetite.

Vitamins & Natural Remedies

Eating natural and wholesome food is necessary to maintain good health. The following powerful vitamins and minerals are found in a variety of healthy foods:

Omega 3 fats:

These heart-friendly fats may lower your risk of heart disease, cancer, dementia, Alzheimer's disease, and depression. They can be found in salmon, trout, sardines, mackerel, and herring.

Calcium & Vitamin D:

Vital for strong bones. Milk is a good source of the mineral calcium and best consumed with Vitamin D that helps the body absorb calcium. Vitamin D can help reduce the risk of some cancers including colorectal cancer. Salmon, yogurt, cheese, and egg yolks are excellent sources of Vitamin D, and so is the sun.

Vitamin C and Vitamin E:

Vitamin C is ascorbic acid that helps your body form collagen needed to make skin, tendons, ligaments, and blood vessels. It is essential for healing wounds and for repairing and maintaining bones and teeth. Vitamin C and vitamin E are known as antioxidants, substances that block some of the damage caused by free radicals created when your body transforms food into energy. Antioxidants may also help prevent cancer and heart disease.

Sources for vitamin C: oranges, apples, kiwi, strawberries, peppers, potatoes, tomatoes. Sources for vitamin E: vegetable oils, wheat germ, nuts, sunflower seeds, leafy greens, papayas, avocadoes. Remember to eat 7-10 servings of fruits and vegetables a day to get your recommended daily dosages of vitamin C (500 mgs) and vitamin E (2 IU).

Magnesium:

Magnesium works with other minerals to relax nerves and relieve tension. It aids digestion and adds alkalinity to body fluids. It promotes sleep and is vital for solid teeth and bones and aids in the metabolism of calcium and vitamin C. Magnesium plays an important part in neuromuscular contractions.

The benefits and whole food sources of vitamins and minerals is health insurance. It is important to supplement our food to ensure our bodies have the proper nutrition to remain healthy. Here is my list of daily supplements to make up any deficiencies in my diet:

> 1 ASA Aspirin 81 mg
> 1 Vitamin E 200 IU
> 1 Vitamin D 600 – 800 IU
> 1 Vitamin C 500 mg (in winter season)
> Calcium 1200 mg
> 3 Glucosamine 500 mg
> No prescription medication = no health problems.

One more thing:

Kick-a-Poo Juice (Blood Purifier)

3 lemons
3 whole heads garlic, peeled

Puree peel, rind and seeds of whole lemons and the garlic
Bring to boil in 3 cups of water. Remove from stove and add
½ cup honey, enough to your taste. Chill. Keep it refrigerated.

Take 2 tablespoons before or after a meal. This tasty elixir will keep for several weeks. It will enhance blood and energy circulation.

Your homework assignment:

Choose healthy foods that you enjoy eating. Plan your grocery list and avoid buying overly processed junk food. Grow some of your food.

> **"If you tickle the earth with a hoe, she laughs with a harvest."**
> — *Douglas William Jarrold*

Be mindful of what you put in your mouth and into your body. Feed your mind and your body with positive thoughts and healthy foods. Moderation is the key. Watch your calorie intake to maintain your optimal weight. Stay away from fad diets.

Discover healthy food choices in your ancestral cuisine. Eat foods that your grandmother would recognize. If you have a multi-cultural background, you have more foods from which to choose. I believe everyone can assemble a good number of the favorite recipes that nourished and nurtured you and your families before you. Make these recipes part of your culinary repertoire.

Eat several small meals a day, every two to three hours. Breakfast is important and eating lunch prevents a lag in energy and a craving for sweets. If you eat only a large meal at night, beware. As a wise Chinese saying goes, "When you eat dinner you feed your enemy."

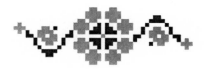

We went to breakfast at a restaurant where the seniors' special was two eggs, bacon, hash browns, and toast for $1.99.

"Sounds good," said my wife. "But I don't want the eggs."

"Then I'll have to charge you two dollars and forty-nine cents because you're ordering a la carte," the waitress warned her.

"You mean I'd have to pay more for not taking the eggs?" my wife asked incredulously. "Yes," replied the waitress.

"Then I'll take the special," my wife said.

"How do you want your eggs?" the waitress asked.

"Raw and in the shell," my wife replied. She took the two eggs home. Don't mess with seniors!

Nine
Secrets of My Success

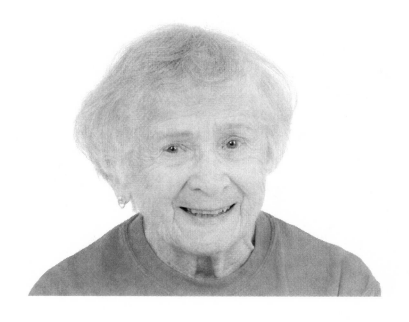

Lesson: Getting old is not for sissies. You have to make up your mind if you want to stay healthy. You have to make the right decisions if you want to be OK as you age. What I do to stay healthy and active has worked for me, and I am sure many of these things may be good for you too. Everyone is different and has a variety of things that energize them. The most important thing to remember is maintaining balance: physical, mental, and emotional. And have fun! Having fun is fundamental.

**"We don't stop playing because we grow old;
we grow old because we stop playing."**
— *George Bernard Shaw*

Imagine that you had won the following prize in a contest: Each morning your bank would deposit $86,400.00 in your private account for your use. However, this prize had rules, just as any game has certain rules. The first set of rules would be: Everything that you didn't spend during each day would be taken away from you.

1. *You may not simply transfer money into some other account.*

2. *You may only spend it.*

3. *Each morning upon awakening the bank opens your account with another $86,400.00 for that day. The second set of rules:*

4. *The bank can end the game without warning, at any time it can say, "It's over, the game is over!"*

5. *It can close the account, and you will not receive a new one.*

What would you personally do? You would buy anything and everything you wanted, right? Not only for yourself but for all people you love, right? Even for people you don't know, because you couldn't possibly spend it all on yourself, right? You would try to spend every cent, and use it all up, right?

Actually this game is Reality.

Each of us is in possession of such a magical bank. We just can't seem to see it. The magical bank is Time.

Each awakening morning we receive 86,400 seconds as a gift of life. And when we go to sleep at night, any remaining time is not credited to us. What we haven't lived up that day is forever lost. Yesterday is forever gone. Each morning the account is refilled, but the bank can dissolve your account at any time . . . without warning.

Well, what will you do with your 86,400 seconds? Aren't they worth so much more than the same amount in dollars? Think about that and always think of this: Enjoy every second of your life because time races by so much quicker than you think. Take care of yourself and enjoy life!

When I first read this unusual, inspiring story its message resonated with me. Time is precious. As you come to the end of my book, you now have a good idea how I spend my daily 86,400 seconds: Exercising, travelling, competing, worshipping, singing, creating, gardening, cooking and volunteering. I recently passed my annual medical exam, and I was able to renew my driver's license. Nowadays, I drive only in the daytime, and I love the independence to drive myself and my friends to our various activities.

And, of course, I love to laugh. When someone asked me the secret to my athletic success I told them, "I don't wear a diaper." Then we both started to laugh. People say I have a healthy sense of humour, and I don't like to disappoint anyone. I hope the jokes that I included in my book brought a smile to your face and tickled your funny bone. Remember, you don't stop laughing because you grow old; you grow old because you stop laughing. Laughter is the best medicine.

Seriously, I do believe the reason I am able to take part in jumping competitions at this advanced age is due to the fact that I have strong muscles and internal organs that are still firmly in place. Our skeletal muscles—the fibres anchored to our bones and tendons that enable both motion and force—are essential to how we function. If we don't take care of these muscles, which can start to deteriorate as young as 25, we are at risk of injury as well as a range of problems from incontinence to weak bones to increased risk for falls—one of the main reasons for reducing lifespan in those over 65.

On November 7, 2012 my strong bones and muscles would be put to an unusual test during my yearly dinner date with my former Glenwood School grade 1 students. What started out as our usually jovial and memorable annual event nearly ended in disaster.

I had anticipated a lovely dinner with Allen Wong and his wife Karen, Cappie Soames, Linda Kelley, Alena Leong, and Marilyn McLennan. As in past years, I knew that there would be lots of laughter and camaraderie as we shared those early childhood memories and adventures. Each of my students had enjoyed different and fulfilling careers, and most of them were now retired. They shared stories of their latest travels, cruise trips, and the exploits of their children and grandchildren.

Dinner, as usual, was delicious. Little did I know that I would be providing the evening's entertainment, the icing on the cake. After collecting our things and arranging my transportation home we proceeded to leave the restaurant. As I prepared to descend the 11 or 12 ceramic steps leading to the front door, I suddenly felt myself start to slip, fall and begin to slide headfirst down the stairs. I was aware I was moving downward, but there was absolutely nothing I could do to catch myself or stop at any point. It didn't take long to get to the bottom. As I glanced up, I could see the look of horror on my students' faces. My audience was appalled and astonished to see my outstretched body on the floor below. I had a smile on my face, and I was talking all the time, as much to calm them as to reassure myself that I was OK.

Cappie was the first one down the stairs. She was trained in First Aid and she made sure I was comfortable and immediately requested an ambulance. She was my Guardian Angel. She noticed a small bump on the right side of my forehead and a bruise, the size of an egg on my left elbow. She secured my neck so that it was stable. In a few minutes the paramedics arrived. They checked my reflexes and awareness, and they escorted me to the Vancouver General Emergency.

What a great, wonderful and competent bunch of medical experts! The emergency doctors checked me over from head to toe with X-rays and scans. To their amazement they determined there were no broken bones. In a few hours, I was able to walk out of the hospital on my own steam, and my son-in-law Richard brought me home at 1:30 a.m. After three Tylenols and my evening prayers I slept until 7:30 a.m. I enjoyed a good breakfast, and only then did I begin to take a good look at my bruised and battered body. No blood.

A bruise the size of an egg on my left elbow meant that was the side on which I sashayed down those 12 hard steps. I was determined that I would be back to normal in a week if not sooner. This was one of the most memorable if horrible moments in my life, especially in front of my students. I hope we will still continue our annual dinners, but I imagine they will choose restaurants on the ground floor. I am so very proud of them.

Before Richard and I left the Vancouver General emergency ward, a doctor showed us an x-ray of my lungs. There was a shadow visible on my right lung. This is being monitored. In the meantime, I will continue to do my deep breathing exercises and reflexology. Who knows how long that shadow has been there?

Two weeks after the nightmare fall, my left hamstring was a horrible dark blue, but my left arm from the wrist to the elbow took the brunt of the fall, and it too was a horrible dark blue. It was swollen and painful.

Do you see the benefits of my daily exercise and stretching routines? Sashaying headfirst down 12 ceramic stairs could have been the end of this 93-year-old. It's amazing, isn't it? Each of us has that seemingly miraculous capacity for regaining health. It's wonderful how the body can heal itself. The key is to be optimistic. This is my mantra: I am active and energetic. I am healthy. I do not get cramps in my legs. I continue to dress standing up. I wash my kitchen and bathroom floors on my hands and knees with a scrub brush. I walk upright with a good stride. No chicken steps or a cane for me, not yet. Thank God.

The main secret I want to share with you is this: You need to think positively and not give in to that side of yourself that wants to mope and stay in bed. I'm so fortunate to be able to do what I love, to perform, and to reach out to so many people. Every day I say affirmations where I wish for good health and positive thinking to get my mind and spirit in the right place. It is important to remind yourself of all the good things in your life—your health, your children, your friends, and your good fortune.

Yes, you will get old. In a culture that is fixated on youth, few people know how to be old. Let me share with you what I have learned over the course of 95 years:

Every day is a gift that we should celebrate

As we age we only get better

You can do anything you set your mind to if you keep reasonable expectations and accept that everything won't go the way you want all the time

Giving up is never an option

Wishing for something won't make it happen; you have to work for it

Focus on the positive and feel good about yourself every day

It's never too late to get fit

Stay in peak physical condition

Adhere to a regimen of a healthy balanced diet and daily exercise

Walk tall, head over shoulders, shoulders over hips

Look ahead and smile

In my experience, happiness and well-being go hand in hand. I applaud the work of our universities, and I have been happy to contribute to the study and research at McGill University and the Beckman Institute. Recently, I read that researchers at San Francisco University who are studying happiness came up with five characteristics of happy people. This is what they discovered: Happy people manage their money well. Happy people spend their money on life experiences rather than material goods. Happy people think fondly about the past and skip over the bad bits. Happy people are empathetic, sharing the happiness and sorrow of others. And lastly, happy people live in communities where they have a sense of belonging, freedom, and of being valued.

The aging population is creating changes, and no doubt there will be challenges. As we face these challenges there will be plenty of reasons to be healthy and happy and celebrate life. One of the hardest things for people in this busy world is to make time for themselves and to put themselves first. Feel confident. Make time for yourself at any age. If you are active now, don't stop even for a week. A basic law in physics states that a body in motion stays in motion. Cherish the 86,400 seconds deposited daily into your daily account.

These days turning 60, 70, 80, and even 90 years of age will be nothing if you take care of yourself, for nothing is beyond a woman or man's reach. Old age isn't a disease any more than infancy. When it comes to health and wellness, seniors are not just part of the problem; we are actually part of the solution. We might even be worth more to the world alive than dead. As Margaret Wilboar, RN, 96 years young said, "Never lose sight of the fact that old age needs so little—but needs that little so much." I see each new year as a gift that I was given to celebrate more time on this planet. We should all feel blessed to grow old. This is the gift of growing older.

Extract and utilize your inner strength for a healthy body, mind, and spirit. Get well and stay well with a healthy mind-set. Mind and spirit are essential to compliment your physical health. Imagery is the language your mind uses to communicate with your body.

Each day thousands of thoughts, images, and sensations flit through our brains as if they were real ones. Imagine and visualize yourself as the best you can be. Engage in the healing process and do your best to help your body heal and remain healthy. I always tell myself, it is never too late to feel good and healthy all over.

Meditate, reflect and contemplate. Meditation has been shown to reduce high blood pressure, headaches, chronic pain, and boost the immune system. Practice meditation daily for 15-20 minutes in a quiet spot, sitting in a comfortable position, taking deep breaths.

When you are aware that your posture is bad, automatically adjust into a more upright energetic position. Good posture is developed through the constant awareness of how you stand, walk, and sleep. When walking or standing hold your head tall, head over your shoulders, shoulders over your hips and hips pushing forward. Look ahead, not down. Swing your arms. Smile!

Approach the problems in your life not with fear but with a healthy sense of curiosity. If you are experiencing an illness do not consider it a punishment. Your body may simply be trying to get your attention. Look for ways to heal. If you are under a doctor's care, put aside your doubts. Be 100% proactive about the treatment. If you have major doubts about your care and treatment, it may interfere with your ability to get well. I believe in yoga. Why are we doing yoga? Yoga means union of mind, body, and spirit.

After an illness, you can help your body recover through the medium of your mind using techniques like meditation, guided visualization, and yoga. Yoga is a gentle, compassionate modality that works with the limits of your body. Yoga poses force blood out of vital organs allowing fresh blood to take its place. This not only cleanses our organs but also provides more nutrients to make our organs stronger and more resistant to disease. Keep the abdominals drawn in and engaged to support the lower back. Yoga poses lengthen your hip flexors, restore the range of motion in your spine, and stimulate your digestive system.

You and I have such valuable resources available to help us get well and stay well with the help of the *The OK Way to a Healthy, Happy Life*. Peace happens when tension leaves your body.

Test your limits and surpass them to achieve goals you never thought possible. It's the little sparkle that lights up your eyes and dances in your smile that makes you gorgeously unique. Greet the day with laughter and enjoy who you are. These are the real beauty and health secrets that never go out of style.

As our age changes, so too does our body. On staying fit, healthy eating must become a lifetime commitment. For pain reduction, improved immunity, strong bones, good balance, and a healthy, sound mind, eat 4–5 small healthy meals a day. I enjoy eating many kinds of nutritious food, only in moderation, and I enjoy a glass of wine with dinner or while watching *Jeopardy*. Red wine is the better alcohol and a good tool against stress that helps us relax. I enjoy a good scotch, now and then, for medicinal purpose only.

Daily supplements of vitamins and minerals as well as glucosamine sulfate for your joints, can fill in for any nutrients that may be missing in your diet. Good food and exercise are your first line of defense and can replace medication. Luckily, more of us are practicing complementary and alternative health care and eliminating prescription drugs. Use common sense and help your body to heal and to take care of itself.

One often finds a lot of tension in the face from frowning or squinting because of eye strain. Raise your eyebrows and open your eyes as wide as possible. At the same time, open your mouth to stretch the muscles around the nose and chin and stick out your tongue. Hold this stretch for 10-15 seconds. Getting the tension out of the muscles in your face will make you smile.

While doing the facial exercises demonstrated in chapter seven, remember to massage the upper gums as you move on the top lip to the ear and the bottom gums moving from the ear to the bottom lip. Gums recede a lot as you age, so keep your gums healthy and strong. As for teeth, flossing daily is one way to stop decay before it starts.

I'd like to share some of my other secrets: when you are brushing your teeth, brush your tongue and along your gums and lips. I dip my toothpaste in a combination of equal parts baking soda and salt for that extra oomph. Rinse well, especially in the morning, so that your mouth will feel squeaky clean and ready to enjoy a good breakfast.

To attack nail fungus I've tried numerous remedies: tea tree oil, balm salve, bleach, vinegar, honey, and lemon zest, with which I was not happy. My latest attempt is applying toothpaste with ginger. I want to believe it is under arrest and not spreading. Open toe shoes don't add to my fashion sense.

I am addicted to Sudoku puzzles. Not that I am so good at it, but I try to solve 2 or 3 that I find in *The Vancouver Sun* and *The Province* newspapers. Since retiring from the Hospital and Homebound teaching, I have been delivering 6 to 7 little booklets of puzzles and games to the children at the Vancouver Children`s Hospital. I compile the booklets from the daily morning comic section.

One of the best vitamins is Vitamin F, which stands for friends, an essential vitamin important for our well-being. Why do we have friends who are all so different in character? How can you get along with all of them? Each one can bring out a different part in us. With one you can be polite. With another friend you can pray.

With another you can laugh and joke. You can sit down and discuss serious matters with another. Your friends are like pieces of a jigsaw puzzle. When completed they form the treasure box, a treasure box of friends. Research shows that people in strong social circles have less risk of depression and terminal strokes. Friends are good for your health. Value your friends and keep in touch with them.

Laugh. A little humour makes life richer and healthier. Research has shown that while engaging in games and sports, it is important to be happy and have fun. Fun contributes to many mental and physical benefits. Endorphins (the body's feel-good chemicals) are released and boost the immune system. Laughter and fun increase creativity, reduce pain and speed healing. Keep an emergency laughter kit that contains funny videotapes, jokes, cartoons, and photographs. Put it with your First Aid supplies and keep it well stocked.

Greet each day with laughter and enjoy who you are. This truly is the best secret that never goes out of style. According to a recent study, happier people make more money. So smiling and laughing is good for your health, your well-being, and your wallet.

Reflect on the nature of beauty as you age. Embrace it and look fabulous. Isn't it wonderful that wrinkles don't hurt! Massaging your face, head and body will rejuvenate the elasticity in your skin and also improve the colour and texture of your hair. Massaging my hair and head has improved the colour of my hair, and my hair is not getting any whiter or grayer.

You will neither need to be lifted nor botoxed. A mind-lift is better than a face-lift. Your thoughts become your words, your words become your actions, your actions become your habits, and your habits become your character. Think positively. Always.

Learn to take control of your health. Love your aging body. It's never too late to achieve optimum health. Good flexibility in your body is crucial to preventing injuries. Therefore, discipline yourself with determination, perseverance, endurance, and honesty—no cheating!

Practice body awareness. At the age of 95, I am aware of my body; I neither ignore it nor resent it. Don't look at your body as a stranger, but adopt a friendly approach toward it. Love your body. Think on this: if you don't know where you are in time and space in this vast universe, how does your immune system know where or how far to go to protect you?

Go to what makes you happy. I love travelling, bowling, athletic competition, fun, and camaraderie. I truly enjoy aquafit plus classes 3 times a week—aerobics in the water at the local swimming pool. Jacuzzi and hot massage feels wonderful. I sit on the edge of the Jacuzzi and put the soles of my feet against the jets for a foot massage. I do reflexology on my hands and feet. Massaging different parts of the foot can stimulate and treat the whole body. Study the reflexology charts included in this book to learn the location of energy channels that connect to the various organs and tissues, and follow my well-developed program.

Self-reflexology on feet and hands done well at home, at your leisure, is in many ways more economical and convenient than having it done in a clinic. I don't encourage people to use reflexology instead of western medicine, but rather as an alternative preventive means to maintain good health, or as a last resort when nothing else works. Reflexology has its limits. It cannot cure cancer or a broken hip. It sends energy to the organs and other parts in the body. I endorse it. Eventually it becomes easier and more convenient to do. Persist.

There are a number of other complementary therapies that you may find useful and want to try. Craniosacral therapy is based on the concept that the bones in the skull are constantly moving, causing the head to expand and contract about 10 times per minute. Manipulating the skull moves the cerebrospinal fluid around the spine and down the sacrum. This in turn manipulates the membranes supporting the brain, resulting in a realignment of the bones so that they resume their natural position and function, enabling the cerebral-spinal fluid to circulate freely. Craniosacral therapy is effective in relieving migraines, tinnitus, dyslexia, eye strain, depression, and chronic pain. This therapy may also help children with brain injuries, slow development, and hyperactivity.

Healing touch is an energy-based therapeutic approach to restore harmony and balance in the body's energy system in order to help the person self-heal. It is a gentle laying on of hands.

Therapeutic touch involves the transfer of life energy through touch, or by holding hands over the affected part of the body. Scientific studies of this form of therapy show that it increases the oxygen-carrying capacity of red blood cells, lowers high temperatures, and reduces restlessness. It has been found particularly effective in treating circulatory lymphatic, musculo-skeletal, and some mental disorders, while alleviating stress in the central nervous system.

Reiki or "universal life-energy" is an ancient oriental energy transfer therapy. Through touch and gentle brushing of the auric field, natural energy flow is restored, which enables us to heal at the physical, emotional, mental, and spiritual levels.

I came across an interesting article that I wish to share with you. Why should we learn the correct procedures to administer CPR (cardiopulmonary resuscitation) to someone who may require it?

Too often we take our hearts for granted. As a mechanical pump, the heart is very reliable and, on average, beats 70 times per minute, which is more than 100,000 times per day. During the average lifetime, the heart beats nearly three billion times and pumps almost five litres of blood per minute, which is over 150 million litres in an average lifetime. The heart pumps blood over 90,000 kilometres of blood vessels. In a fraction of a second, this can change when a person suffers a heart attack or goes into cardiac arrest. Learn how to perform CPR and you may save someone's life.

The simplest procedures can bring the greatest results. After shopping, or before a competition, I elevate my feet 45° angle for at least 30 minutes. I even doze off, which tells me that my body needed rejuvenation. If I do this while watching *Jeopardy*, I often miss out on the winners.

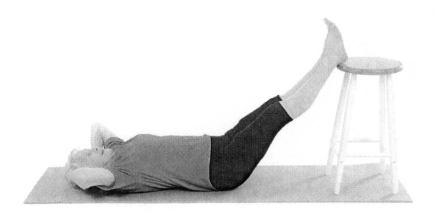

I believe I have been blessed with high energy and good genes. As someone said, genes may load the gun, but lifestyle pulls the trigger. The only time in my life when I experienced some anxiety and needed recuperation was after three changes to my body: the birth of my two daughters, a hysterectomy, and a tooth extraction. These instances were relatively mild compared to what others have suffered; yet, it would have been easy for me to slip into ill health if I did not work hard at staying fit.

Sometimes in the middle of the night when nature calls, and you must get up to go to the bathroom, if you find you still can't fall back to sleep, don't curse your insomnia. Take advantage of this time to do the routine stretching exercises in bed as I have described in this book. Your house will be quiet; the phone won't ring. Rather than get upset that you can't fall back to sleep, make use of this precious time. My stretching exercises performed for 90 minutes three times a week have sustained me for years, and I know that they will sustain you too.

Concentrate on each stretch as you count reps without any interruptions. Remember to hold each stretch for 30 seconds. Start your facial and head massage while simultaneously holding a belt to stretch your legs. As I mentioned above, facial and body muscle exercises have even improved my hair colour. Deep breathing and elevating your feet at 45 degrees for ½ hour are equally important.

Manipulate the muscles in your arms, shoulders, torso, and legs with your thumbs and palms ending in the solar plexus (the pit of the stomach). Incorporate the use of sponge balls. Stretch out your whole body. Oxygenate your body by deep breathing (in through the nose, count 1-4 rest and out through the mouth count 5-10) ten times minimum. Your body will be exhilarated. When was the last time you felt your own back? Massage your whole body. Love your body.

Sleep is important. Get your 7-8 hours every night. Beauty sleep is for real. You will look better. Sleep can prevent dark circles, bloodshot eyes, and sallow complexion. When you are sleep deprived not only do you look fatigued but you look less attractive. I try to sleep as much as possible. I work all the time. I don't go to bars or restaurants. I don't party. I doze off while reading the morning newspaper while eating breakfast after aquafit. After my routine stretching exercises at night, I easily fall asleep again, no tossing or turning, and sleep for another 3-4 hours without interruptions. I am told that I snore, but luckily I don't hear myself! I sleep alone.

Staying active can help you keep your independence and manage symptoms of illness, prevent falling, and maintain good balance and strong health. The rewards of exercise and sports are immeasurable. Thus, I want to educate people to do regular physical exercises. Health is the most treasured possession we have.

My adopting an athletic lifestyle as a senior suggests that it is possible to improve speed, strength, and power later in life. My life proves that it's never too late to start, even if you didn't acquire strong athletic skills as a youngster. Ironically, I may have benefitted from the fact that I didn't take part in strenuous athletics as a young woman: I may have been a candidate for a hip or knee replacement.

As a youngster, I worked hard on the farm in the early morning fresh air and sunshine before trekking off to school with my brothers and sisters. Now, I am not saying that you should move to the country and take up farming, unless you want to, but your new morning routine can mean waking up early to a light breakfast, taking a brisk walk for one hour in the fresh morning air, and combining your walk with deep-breathing exercises.

If you have a garden, spend a few hours in moderate physical labour. There is something spiritual and invigorating about working in a garden—fresh air, birds, bees, bugs, flowers, vegetables. This past summer, after working in my garden, digging, raking, and planting for hours, my body was naturally tired. I listen to my body. Although I think I would like to work a little bit longer, my body says that's enough. I go into the house for a cup of tea. While resting my legs against the wall for ½ hour or more, or watching TV, doing a Sudoku, reading the newspaper, my body enjoys the rest and relaxation. In another hour or so, I feel relaxed and ready to move again. My muscles are rested and repaired at that time; therefore, I believe regular massaging helps and enables my body to repair and to become energized faster.

Here are my genuine suggestions for a healthy and happy life:

Exercise daily. A balance of hard/easy routines works for me, alternating 3 days of strength training exercises with 3 days of aerobic exercises.

Eat only wholesome food and avoid junk foods.

Drink plenty of water.

Enjoy getting out in nature: garden and make things grow.

Connect with family, friends, and community.

Discover what you truly like to do and try to do it as often as possible. Do what makes you happy.

Do something nice for yourself.

Take a nap without feeling guilty.

Hard to get started?

Start today. Exercise daily and moderately for two weeks and then gradually increase your activity level with conviction and perseverance. You will learn ways to feel energetic, vibrant, and alive while still feeling content, calm, and peaceful. When you use your body in different ways you become stronger and fitter.

30-60 minutes of moderate physical activity

20 – 30 minutes, rigorous activity like brisk
walking, hiking, dancing, aerobics, jogging,
swimming, aqua fit—relax, retreat, rejuvenate

3 x week, muscle strengthening activities
Gym, weights, working in the garden

Reflexology on feet and hands

Yoga

Here is my personal recipe to keep you looking and feeling young from inside out:

Daily diet should consist of plenty of
fruits and vegetable for the vitamins,
minerals, and fiber they contain.

Maintain an alkaline high carbohydrate,
low protein, low bad fat diet.

Watch your salt and sugar intake.
Use honey and herbs.

Protect your skin—drink lots of
water, at least 3 litres daily.

Keep your heart from aging; eat
salmon and other fish.

Protect your brain from dementia with
fruits, vegetables, and mind games.

Take vitamins C,D,E and calcium.

Eat lean proteins, meat, beans, and whole grains.

Take 1 baby aspirin a day.

To repeat: The magic ingredients for
maintaining weight—fiber, protein, water.

Your muscles stretch more easily when your body is properly hydrated. Drink plenty of Water—8 glasses a day. Relaxed stretches help your body function more naturally and allow you to sleep more soundly. Take your time, stretch with control, and breathe deeply. For optimal performance, I drink water before, during, and after workouts. Water is the fountain of youth: it keeps our skin clear, hair shining, energy high, and weight within the healthy range. Forget about expensive anti-aging creams. Water keeps skin wrinkle-free longer. Go get a glass of water right now. It may be all you need to boost how you look and perform.

Walking is the best exercise and does not require any special talent or apparatus except for a pair of good walking shoes. Keep your head over your shoulders, shoulders over hips, pushing forward. Look ahead not down. Let your feet do the walking. Swing your arms. When you are aware that your posture is bad, automatically adjust into a more upright, energetic position. Good posture is developed through the constant awareness of how you sit, stand, walk, and sleep.

It's been said that if you walk a mile a day every day without increasing your calorie intake you could lose 10 pounds of fat in one year. Smile and enjoy the fresh air, sunshine, and singing birds. Be happy. If you are active now, don't stop even for one week. Remove any barriers. Getting older is no excuse to slow down! Develop self-esteem and confidence. Be proud of yourself. Life is too grand and too short to set up barriers. Just get out there and do it. There is so much energy, so much excitement, so many possibilities waiting for you. All you have to do is wake up and look.

Late in life, I found I loved track and field, which allowed me to travel around the world meeting many new people. I found the *Fountain of Youth* in a swimming pool. As an athlete I try to escape the bounds of gravity by running, jumping, and throwing things. It may have something to do with that bump on the road on the way to my baptism. Who knows? Life is a funny blend of destiny, chance, and choice, and there will be some things we can't change, so we have to accept them and move on. If we can determine the course of events, we must choose life. I choose to be healthy, happy, and alive to my very last breath.

I also believe that we should stay happy, healthy and, yes, even sexy! We don't lose interest in sex because we get old; we get old because we lose interest in being attractive, appealing, and approachable. Looking positive and attractive, and feeling healthy and strong will definitely help us achieve our goals in sports and athletics with much fun and anticipation.

Have more fun. Why is having fun so important to us? Frequent bouts of fun have a host of proven mental and physical benefits. Having fun relieves stress and triggers the release of endorphins (the body's feel-good chemicals). It helps boost the immune system.

We need to engage our body in forms of play and games to get rid of stress that we encounter every day. Go for a walk on a bright sunny day, enjoy the scenery, smell the flowers, and return home newly energized. When people have fun they get inspired positively. The theory is that fun can change people's behavior for the better.

Learn to manage your energy. Master your will and honour the rhythm of life. Someone asked me how I manage to travel around the world to various sports' competitions, sometimes alone, negotiating my way around enormous airports. I confess that sometimes I ask for a wheelchair when transferring from one terminal to another. So, the next time you see an elderly person sitting in an airport wheelchair, don't pity them. They just may be conserving their vital energy to compete at a master's athletics championship.

The film industry is recognizing that the population is aging, and they have created some interesting films. I highly recommend the following movies.

Quartet. "You're never too old for love." This film follows four elderly 80-year-old musicians and singers who live and love in a senior's residence.

Autumn Gold. "You're never too old for athletics, sport and track & field." This German documentary features five elderly athletes, 80 to 100 years old, doing track and field. The film crew follows them as they prepare for the 2009 WMA Championships in Lahti, Finland. I am featured in the film when I meet Gabre Gabrc, a Croatian-born Italian track and field athlete who was born in 1917 and competed in the 1936 summer Olympics.

Ping Pong. "You're never too old for ping-pong." This documentary from England features eight, elderly table-tennis players who prepare for and compete in a ping pong championship. The movie is humorous, entertaining, and encouraging.

Every day, I am thankful to have my health and strength to be able to stay active, contribute to the world, to my community, to be with my family and friends, and to live life to the fullest. It is the health of our body, mind, and spirit that is the foundation of each and every community. It builds pride. I wholeheartedly support the promotion of sports by our energetic and spirited senior athletes, and I hope my book will be a catalyst to those who want to venture into this area of activity.

Growing up with my ten brothers and sisters on the farm in Saskatchewan, I never imagined that almost 100 years later I would be doing what I am doing now. After retiring from a job I loved, I didn't want to just sit around and not be challenged. On the contrary, at the age of 77 I became entranced by track and field. I chose to become a young-at-heart athlete rather than an old woman. I always wanted to feel young and capable, be healthy and vibrant and yes, even sexy! I have just turned 95 and I intend to keep smelling the roses for some time to come, God willing.

As you come to the end of my book, I have a confession to make. I have come to realize that when you start reminiscing about the past, that's when you start aging. I don't do nostalgia. I don't do guilt. I have a really stable life, and I am much more giving and less quick to judge.

Despite my accomplishments, I feel my personal success in a vulnerable way. Why? Because I don't feel I deserve it. I've never had such a feeling before in my life. Where is it coming from? So, who's OK? I don't know. I once was Frances, and then I became Olga. I've been a daughter, sister, aunt, teacher, wife, mother, grandmother, friend, and traveller. In my later years, I became Olga the athlete. We know that the body regenerates itself many times throughout a life of activity and rest. We know, as we age, the mind learns, forgets, and learns again. We also know that in our quiet moments we can sense our spirit mature. All these changes affect our identity as strongly as our cultural heritage, our genetics, and our personality. We are never a static being, locked into our circumstances; we can alter our existence and take on new challenges at any stage of life. In March of 2014, I will be 95. Maybe I haven't quite caught up to myself as a 95-year-old athlete. Maybe I still see myself as a little girl happy to play baseball, or a young woman enthusiastic to teach. I don't know. So, who's OK? As a life-long learner, I hope I have a number of years ahead of me to answer that question.

When I told a friend that I started to have serious doubts about the value of writing this book, she suggested I read an inspiring speech by a 94-year-old, South African President Nelson Mandela:

> **"Our deepest fear is not that we are inadequate. Our deepest fear is that we are powerful beyond measure. It is our light, not our darkness, that most frightens us. We ask ourselves, who am I to be brilliant, gorgeous, talented, fabulous? Actually, who are you not to be? You are a child of God. Your playing small doesn't save the world. There's nothing enlightened about shrinking so that other people won't feel insecure around you. We are all meant to shine, as children do. We were born to make manifest the glory of God that is within us. It's not just in some of us; it's in everyone. And as we let our own light shine, we unconsciously give other people permission to do the same.**

As we're liberated from our own fears, our presence automatically liberates others."

South Africa's first black president, Nelson Mandela, passed away in December 2013. If he had not been imprisoned for 27 years he may have lived to be well over 100. As it was, despite all of the pain and indignities that he endured, Mandela lived to the age of 95. Africans are proud to say that he was Africa's greatest gift to the world. I believe that. He taught the world that we can only survive and thrive if we truly forgive those who have hurt us. When we forgive, we make a concerted effort to let go of a grudge. We recognize human frailty and fallibility and embrace our common humanity.

Mandela also believed that education is the most powerful weapon that you can use to change the world. I aim to continue learning and developing my talents to their fullest and to stay consistent with them until I know or realize that it's time to ease up and eventually stop. At the moment I have no intention to stop or even hesitate. I still have the energizer in action that keeps me healthy and active.

After giving it some thought, I have decided that upon my death I will leave my body to medical science with the hope that by doing so I can continue teaching even after I am gone. Perhaps a scientist will unlock the secret of my energy—physical, mental, and spiritual. Where does this energy come from?

Our body, mind, and spirit are constantly interrelating. This action produces the power that creates harmony and balance in our life. Body is physical, mind is mental, and spirit is emotional and spiritual. I arrived at this conclusion. I believe that my stamina, courage, tenacity, mental strength, and optimistic spirit come from my Christian faith. My parents set an amazing foundation for that faith. For me, my faith is very personal, and it is consistent with my desire to make a difference in the world.

Faith, prayer, and spiritual beliefs play an important role in our lives, and in our health. As a Christian, I believe that everything happens for a purpose and that God guides and directs us. So, when adversities and tests cross my path, I pay attention and question whether this direction is the one I am supposed to take. There is a certain self-confidence, clarity of purpose and, most important, generosity of spirit combined to accomplish the task at hand. Have faith in God. Trust God, and all will be well. I see how the body cannot be alone without the mind and spirit. Spiritual nourishment comes when I receive the body and blood, soul and divinity of Jesus Christ (the bread and wine) in the sacrament of the Holy Eucharist.

I am a firm believer that meditation and relaxation energize the internal benefits of quietude, peace, and a sense of well-being. All my life, I have been active in the Ukrainian community promoting the spiritual traditions and customs according to the Ukrainian Catholic Church. The fundamental aim of the Catholic faith is to develop, enrich, and preserve the religious and spiritual life. I am proud of my faith and my dedication to the spiritual aspects of life.

Thank you, Lord, for my 95-year-old healthy body, mind, and spirit. God willing, there will be many more championships in track and field to come. My life has certainly been enriched, and I feel blessed. I believe the Holy Spirit guides me in all my endeavours. My mind and heart remain intrinsically linked to the many individuals who gave me so much of what is precious to me today. I pray for my family and for my many wonderful friends all over the world.

I believe and I quote Oprah Winfrey's belief in spirituality: "It isn't until you come to a spiritual understanding of who you are—not necessarily a religious feeling, but deep down, the spirit within—that you can begin to take control." During "An Evening with Oprah Winfrey" on January 24, 2013 at the Rogers Arena in Vancouver, an ecstatic 16,000 strong audience embraced the influential, media icon. Winfrey talked about "listening to your inner voice", whether you consider it the voice of God or as she likes to say "your emotional GPS on the road to self-realization".

We enjoyed the wisdom, favourite stories, and the candour of Oprah. "No matter what you are struggling through, no matter the pain or anguish, you can go inside behind your mind and observe it happening to you. When you come to know this, you realize that even though the canvass of your life is painted with daily experiences, behaviours, and emotions, you are the one controlling the brush."

My secret: Stop. Rest. Find a few moments in the day to close your mind to the outside world, nurture your spirit, mind, and body and restore your peaceful energy. Count your blessings. Everyone has some.

I believe I reconnect with the Spirit that nurtures the human soul and, thereby, my stress is reduced, and a powerful energy is restored. This is my personal belief. I listen for the soft, gentle voice of my heart and soul, the voice of trust and justice, and the beat of my life as it rejuvenates.

I truly feel a strong bond with my Lord, and He has always blessed me with wonderful experiences. I am so thankful for the gifts given to me by my Lord. My faith has helped me stay motivated enough to be healthy and compete in track and field from the age of 77 to 95.

Thank you, my Lord, for my wonderful parents, sisters, brothers, children, grandchildren, and friends.

I will continue to contribute and support wherever it is needed. I will try to exemplify, teach, and encourage seniors as well as children of all ages to challenge themselves and to contribute to their community. I believe each one of us, especially seniors, has the physical, mental, and spiritual potential to enjoy recreation, sport, and healthy living and, thereby, not burden our health care system. You and I have such valuable resources to help us get well and stay well with the help of *The O.K. Way to a Healthy, Happy Life*. We must be determined to run the race that is ahead of us.

When the time comes, and it certainly will for me to retire and stop competing in track and field, I hope to take piano lessons. That old piano should again resonate in the house. As well, I will buy a computer to join the contemporary mood of the crowd. I do have a golf club and some balls. Who knows how this physical activity of my life will serve me. I should keep on being vibrant and profitable to my community.

It is my sincere hope that this book will be a catalyst to help seniors, and people of all ages, to start improving their health through daily exercise, good food, community activity, and a gratitude to the Heavenly Creator. In my daily prayers, I include the welfare of my family and all of my friends. Each morning, remember to be grateful for what the world brings to you. Say your prayers tonight and express that gratitude.

French woman Jeanne Calment, who was the world's oldest woman since her date of birth could be verified, passed away at 122 years of age. She was an artist and actress and last acted in a movie at the age of 100. Sadly, she and I shared the same heartbreaking experience of losing a daughter to illness at an early age.

Somehow we got through it. When Jeanne was asked the secret behind her longevity she replied: "olive oil, a sense of humour and the fact that I fear nothing."

I plan to follow in her fearless footsteps, and I would like to enjoy another thirty years, to love life and not fear aging. I don't lie about my age. Someone told me that everyone needs a feisty and healthy grandmother from the prairies to remind them what really matters in a complicated world. I am a grandmother who loves to travel around the world, meet new people, and compete. There are plenty of reasons to be healthy and happy and to celebrate life. Today, I have more energy, more strength, more stamina, and more spirit, and I feel great. I have a magnificent life, and I know you can too. It's amazing! I'm loving every minute of it.

I would like to end my book with *The Optimist Creed,* the philosophy of Optimists International. This service club was established in 1911 in Buffalo New York, and it is dedicated to community involvement, in particular to assisting youth in need. There are more than 3000 Optimist clubs worldwide; I belong to the Optimist Club of the North Shore, Vancouver. I hope these words will inspire and support you on this wonderful journey that we call life. This is the most important homework I am assigning.

May the grace of our Saviour Jesus Christ bring you and your loved ones His peace, joy, and love now and forever and ever. Yours faithfully in our Lord, *Olga*.

THE OPTIMIST CREED

Promise yourself:

To be so strong that nothing can disturb your peace of mind

*To talk health, happiness, and prosperity to every person
you meet*

*To make all of your friends feel there is something
in them*

*To look at the sunny side of everything and make your
optimism come true*

*To think only of the best, to work only for the best,
and expect only the best*

*To be just as enthusiastic about the success of others
as you are about your own*

*To forget the mistakes of the past and press on to the
greater achievements of the future*

*To wear a cheerful countenance at all times and give
every living creature you meet a smile*

*To give so much time to the improvement of yourself that
you have no time to criticize others*

*To be too large for worry, too noble for anger, too strong
for fear, and too happy to permit the presence of trouble*

It seems that my life has consisted of multifaceted experiences taking place predominantly in the 21st century. It was a multi-purpose time of learning, growth, and maturing. What did I learn? Be brave. Be different. Don't just take the way things have always been—be the way it has to be. Make your space and add new ideas. Connect with your body.

Life is a game. Play to win.

"Failure is simply the opportunity to begin again this time more intelligently."

— *Henry Ford*

I hope that you will do the homework. My secrets are not secrets anymore because I like to share.

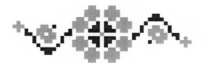

Accolades

Olga is a phenomenon, rarely encountered by most of us as we go through life. For those of us approaching the ripe age of 70 the thought of any human being beginning an "athletic career" at age 77 and commencing to compete not in one's back yard but internationally for the world to see, is beyond comprehension! The entire scenario is even more unbelievable when you learn that Olga, before retiring, was not overly athletically minded nor did she have any strong sports ambitions. Bowling was the closest she came, and that was more for social diversion rather than athletics.

Walter Zavadell
VP Sales & Marketing (retired)

Beyond her incredible athletic feats, Olga is a model of active aging. She travels by herself to seek competitive opportunities (however rarely) against women in her age group. She also takes an interest in the governance of her sport. In Lahti, Finland she observed the General Assembly elections of World Masters Athletics. Olga is a hero to her fellow athletes as well, including world class performers such as Karla Del Grande, who wrote on my site: "Olga is truly inspiring and a real dynamo! Imagine competing in events where no one at the age of 90 has competed before!"

Kenneth Stone
Founder mastertrack.com

As a former teacher, principal and assistant superintendent in the Burnaby School District, I have known Olga as a teacher for many of the thirty-four years that she taught. Throughout her teaching career, Olga demonstrated the kind of commitment that she now demonstrates in her athletic career. I became aware of Olga's second career two years ago when Olga made a presentation at a large luncheon meeting of our association. The presentation was an outstanding success. Our members were in awe of Olga's accomplishments. Olga's athleticism has benefitted her health and overall well-being. Olga definitely practices what she preaches. She encourages the older generation to become stimulated and active in order to enjoy a richer, healthier life. Therefore, changing how we live is Olga's philosophy.

Gerry Dittrich,
President
Burnaby Retired Teachers Association

Olga not only represents the values and aspirations kindred to sport, personal improvement, dedication and hard work, but she has set an outstanding precedent in terms of setting the bar of performance beyond what was currently imagined. This accomplishment has not only set a standard but has pushed the envelope of the possibilities that has been both an inspiration and motivation for others. In Olga's words, "Aging may be affected by our genes, but our real biological age depends largely on our daily habits, stress level and mental and physical exercise." Olga sets that example not only for seniors but also for all of us by participating in activities that contribute to a well-rounded, fit and healthy individual. Olga Kotelko could not have accomplished all this without the one major ingredient that ensures success, and that is attitude. Upon meeting Olga you are immediately aware of her energy and enthusiasm for life portrayed by her positive attitude.

Ralph J. Ferstay
Recreation Service Manager
West Vancouver Parks & Community Service

Olga is a gracious winner. Because of her dedication, determination and talent, her character seldom faces the test of failure. I have only seen her "fail" once. On the third and final day of competition in the North American, Central American and Caribbean Regional Championships in Leon, Mexico at altitude in extreme heat, while running the 200m, she stumbled and fell. She responded by picking herself up and, sporting a scraped and swollen upper lip, readjusted her glasses and went off to compete in and win the weight pentathlon. She is a sweet, young octogenarian, but she is also a fierce competitor. Olga is an inspiration for me and has altered by perspectives. One of my personal goals, now, is to set the world record in the decathlon for men 100+. It may not be easy to do. I suspect I will have competition. Olga has changed the expectations and dreams of many.

Warren Hamill
World Champion, M55 decathlon

It seems that now, in 2012, motivation and inspiration becomes harder to find. It is much easier for kids these days to play on the computer rather than focusing on working hard at something, learning or physical activity. I am here to inform you of one amazing woman who inspires me. Her name is Olga Kotelko.

Olga started competing in shot put, discus and javelin in 1997, and was immediately successful. She then expanded her interests to include 100m, 200m, hammer throw, high jump and pentathlon. Olga has won medals in every event she has participated. In addition to her outstanding athletic achievements, Olga encourages and motivates others about health and fitness. She makes presentations to seniors' groups. She is an active member of the Optimist Club, where she serves as Chairperson of the Youth Sports Committee. She has represented Canada and British Columbia in numerous international track and field competitions.

Olga is an inspiration to every athlete, young and senior, proficient or beginner.

Her dedication and attitude embody the best principles of amateur athletic competition.

Kenneth M. Dawson,
President Optimist Club of the North Shore

———————

The following tributes mean so much to me as I perceive myself through the eyes of my family. Some of their thoughts are serious and some of them are funny but all of them are filled with love.

———————

Mom has a great deal of love and wisdom that she never hesitates to share with any of us. Her love nurtures us and her wisdom binds us together. She knows that by challenging us with hard work, she can help to give us, as individuals, a sense of purpose by binding us together as a family. She gives us a sense of belonging. She creates balance and joy in our lives and has taught us to always strive to make the best of ourselves.

Without Olga's imagination, boldness and boundless energy and curiosity, she would not have become the woman that she is today. Anyone who has worked with her can truly appreciate the range of her talents. We have and we do.

She is ageless, adventurous, active, beautiful, balanced, blessed, charismatic, creative, capable, dynamic, determined, enthusiastic, exuberant, feisty, faithful, flexible, full of life, grateful, genuine, gutsy, hardworking, honest, happy, imaginative, influential, jovial, kind, knowledgeable, loving, motivational, natural, never late, noticeable, optimistic, observant, original, perceptive, poised, persistent, quirky, resilient, reliable, radiant, has stamina, is special, spiritual, trustworthy, thoughtful, unique, vibrant, valuable, versatile, whimsical, wise and forever youthful. Olga is one of a kind. Quite a gal!

Lynda Rabson,
Daughter

As Grandma's most attractive, successful, witty and all round best grandchild I am sorry that I cannot be in Vancouver to share in the experience of her turning 90. Although I am at school over 4500 kilometres away, her life is still very much a part of mine. I am constantly reminded of her every time I turn on a T.V. and see something about the upcoming Olympics, or see the oval track at my school (athough covered by 4 feet of snow for the better part of the year). I feel a great sense of pride when I tell stories about her athletic accomplishments, and I enjoy seeing the baffled faces of my friends when I do.

The lessons she has taught me over the years resonate with me to this day. The virtues of hard work and determination that were ingrained in her from a young age have been imparted to me through many stories about her childhood and the way she carries herself. I feel that she has been an immense part of developing the person that I am today.

Her selfless acts remind me to act ethically in all situations (often difficult at business school), and the kindness and respect that she gives to everyone she meets are unparalleled. I aspire to one day be as well liked as she is, which she accomplishes by being genuine and loving with everyone she meets. And she makes good pyrogies. Thank you Grandma OK.

Matt Rabson,
Grandson

―――――――――

Most of you know my grandmother as the one-in-a-million strong-hearted world athlete, but I'll bet you've never caught onto her secret plan to replicate herself.

Grandma has lived with us since before I was born, and I've caught onto a series of events that lead me to believe that she is trying to turn me into her. I'm not crazy! It's true.

Through my years in pre-school, I would come home after school and Grandma would always be there. Every day after school would be the same. We would take the same red checkered blanket, a bowl of watermelon, and a Ukrainian book, and we would go to the same place on the lawn and she would teach me to read and speak Ukrainian. From what I remember as a 4 year-old, I wasn't half bad. We must have spent hours upon hours outside, slowly learning the nouns and family members (of which I remember baba and gido). I was just having fun, but I was learning her language as well.

As I continued to elementary school, school began to take up more of my time. The afternoon watermelon-Ukrainian lessons slowed down and stopped. We began a new tradition. Every year around Easter, she would put out this array of dyes on the table with wax and candles, and every day, before and after school—because I couldn't get enough of it—we would sit at the table making pysanka. She would tell me the meaning of all the dyes as I put my egg into them and then we would sit and watch the oven apprehensively as the wax would melt off and I could see my final product. All year I would look forward to spending this tradition with her.

Nearing the end of elementary school and into high school, it was discovered that I enjoyed being just as involved with athletics as Gramma is. This led me to join my school's track and field team in grade 4, and I continued through until my grade 12 year. Gramma took the time while I was in elementary school to become the shot put coach of the school team, and even though we had a teacher as coach in high school, I still insisted that she be my personal trainer. At least a couple of afternoons per week, Gramma would take the time away from her own training, and we would head over to the track so that I could practice my throws. I never became a world-class athlete, but finally in my last year in high school we made it to the B.C. provincial championships.

To recap, over the years she has taught me her language, her culture, and got me interested in her sports. There seems to be a pattern here; she has slowly been making me like her.

For this, I have to say thank you, for all the time we've spent together and everything I've learned from you. I hope I can be able to pass down Gramma's kindness, generosity, and love for her family to my own family when I have one of my own.

Alesa Rabson,
Granddaughter

My earliest recollection of Aunty Olga was when I was around five or six years old. The family held her in high esteem as she was the most educated member of the family. She became a teacher, got married to a handsome man named John and then moved away. Later when the marriage ended and she arrived in British Columbia to make a new life for herself and her girls, I was often asked to babysit, and I learned how to change diapers with baby Lynda.

In 1959 she bought a house that was being built by students in New Westminster and had it moved to a lot three doors down from us. She hired people to dig a basement and relatives and neighbours built the forms for the walls and poured the cement. She worked alongside all of us and we learned about building houses and about Olga. Although she encountered many problems to solve and decisions to make while managing different people during the stressful project, I never saw her angry or distressed. She was always open to opinions before she made a decision.

I have stayed in touch with Aunt Olga over the years and she continues to amaze me. Although many of her siblings lived well into their 80's, she has surpassed them all. Hard work is the secret behind her success. She works hard at staying healthy.

As I photographed her demonstrating her exercise routine I realized that her posture has actually improved over the years. It only proves that with awareness, diligence and perseverance, as she likes to say, we can improve our health and well-being no matter what our age. Our birthdays might come and go but Aunty Olga's are precious to us. I wish her many more years of athletic supremacy.

Noris Burdeniuk,
Nephew

The word "hero" means different things to different people. Some people believe that a hero is someone who has changed the world, someone who has changed politics or even someone who has invented something. I agree with all of these things however I wanted to choose someone who is personal to me, someone who could open my eyes and prove to me that they could achieve things I never thought they could. My Aunty Olga did just that.

Olga Kotelko is a track and field athlete. She has traveled around the world participating in competitions, she trains for the 100m, 200m, 400m, shot put, javelin and high jump. She's a busy lady. Actually one day I asked her if there was a track and field event she didn't compete in. She just laughed and said, "Well actually Kelli, there is pole vault but I'm planning to attempt it soon!"

This may not shock you that a person can be in almost every event that track and field has to offer, some of you do it every spring. But the thing that separates my aunty from you is that she is 82 years old. This amazes me because when I picture an 82-year-old I see a small, fragile baba. And when I see my aunty I still see My Great Aunty Olga who is shorter than me and weighs less than I do but in a matter of seconds she could kick my behind.

Aunty Olga has confidence. A lot of confidence. She comes up to a challenge and believes in herself so much that whatever she was planning to accomplish is almost too scared to fight back. And this is one of the reasons she's my hero. She's always been tough. She had to be; she grew up in the 1920s and you'll never guess where her hometown was. It was Smuts, Saskatchewan. She had several daily chores that she split up with her 10 siblings. This is where she learned determination and strength, both physical and mental. She also was a big softball player. She and her friend were the only girls on the local team. They had to walk 6 miles to the game, play and walk 6 miles back home.

When Aunty Olga grew up she moved to Vancouver, where she is currently living. She played softball up to the age of 77 and then moved her talent to track and field by accident. She asked the high school if she could use their equipment, and that was the start of the 77-year- old athletic star. She found a trainer and began practicing for high jump, but that wasn't good enough either. She learned more about track and field events, and she decided to try almost every kind of sport. Currently in 2000 at the age of 81, she has 81 medals in 81 events, which I may add, are all gold. She had also broken world records in discus and javelin and because competition in her age category is hard to find she is challenging herself to break those records again. She has traveled to Australia, Europe, the United States and all over Canada participating in athletic competitions. She believes the unthinkable can be accomplished. I believe she is a Canadian hero because she has the power to change what Canadians think, and she is my hero because she is my auntie. She has shown that determination and dedication can take you anywhere even at the age of 82. And I believe being a track athlete at this age is a great accomplishment because I don't know how many 82-year-olds can even run a meter without breaking a hip. So in closing I would like to thank my Aunty Olga for influencing me and I hope you now see her as a hero too.

Kelli Malko,
Niece

We grew up on a farm in Saskatchewan about 100 kilometres northeast of Saskatoon. Olga was the seventh of eleven children, five boys and six girls. The year Olga was born, dad built our two-storey home with three bedrooms upstairs and three rooms downstairs. The whole house was heated by a small tin heater in the middle of the room downstairs. Of course, we had to double up or triple up when we went to sleep. But we had goose down quilts for covers to keep us warm.

Times were tough. During the dirty 30s I remember when dad went to Smuts for some fish that was offered as relief as we were kind of skimping on food. Towards spring, mom would preserve the fish that were not consumed during the winter in jars. She would fill the jars with fish, bones and all. It was delicious. Mom would also save potato peelings and planted them in spring for a new crop. We all survived and grew up to be adults.

We attended Riel Dana School that was 2 miles away. The first half mile was uphill. At recess we played baseball. For some reason I had to run to the bases as Olga was up to bat. I started to run as she raised the bat upwards and struck me over the eyebrow, where a scar remains to this day.

I was so proud of Olga because she was the first one of the family to attend high school. She boarded with the Sister Servants and attended Bedford Road Collegiate in Saskatoon. She graduated and then attended the Business College and later Teachers College which was then called the Normal School. She taught school in Saskatchewan and later in British Columbia.

Olga was always glamorous, slight, prim and proper. I was a little jealous, as I was pudgy and plain. After Olga married John Kotelko they had their first baby, Nadine, who was their pride and joy. I was privileged to be her godmother. Later on, another bundle of joy, Lynda was born.

Olga always excelled in anything that she did. At an early age she learned to knit and crochet, and she was always good at art. She always kept busy. And we all know that she took up athletic endeavors when she turned 77 years old and she hasn't' stopped yet. She has won hundreds of gold medals in shot put, high jump, running, often breaking her own records.

Olga has proved that where there is a will there is a way, and you can achieve whatever you set your heart on. We are proud of you for being a role model for us, and God bless you for many years of health and happiness.

Phyllis Gutiw,
Sister

(The last of my siblings died on
November 12, 2011 at the age of 88.)

Acknowledgements

It has been said that it takes a community to make a child. Judging from the list that follows the same can be said for writing a book. So many people offered their suggestions, contributions, and support in one way or another to make this book possible. I extend my sincere thanks to all the brilliant minds who took precious time out of their already overbooked days and nights to give their generous support. I hope none are excluded.

I have benefitted immensely over the years from the support and love from my incredible daughter Lynda and son-in-law Richard. Lynda's invaluable assistance deserves special mention because without her this book would have been a much weaker version of itself. She has always been gracious in allowing me to lean on her in many situations, and the book was no different: she was available to help me on short notice whenever I imposed on her time. Both Lynda's and Richard's expert advice, guidance, and encouragement were crucial to making the book the best it could be. Lynda's contribution to the success of this book is immeasurable: she carefully concentrated on dates and details, and kept me on task. I am grateful for her intelligence and kindness. Thank you, Lynda.

My two grandchildren, Matthew and Alesa. You have kept me grounded and added joy and humour to my life. I am so proud of you both and can never thank you enough for your love and support.

I am truly grateful to Roxanne Davies who masterminded the book project from its inception to conclusion. She carefully developed the first draft from my handwritten scribbles and has continued to help to the end. Her faith in the project made it a reality.

North Shore writer/editor Michele Carter polished my story into a shiny and readable narrative that has brought the nine chapters to life. Thank you! www.indiescribbler.com.

A special acknowledgement goes to Andrea Argyros, a prominent West Vancouver artist who has painted several beautiful paintings of me and who suggested the title, *Olga*.

Romy Ilich created a beautiful cover that captures the spirit of my story. http://www.romyilich.com.

I want to thank members of the media who have taken a chance on me and made my story a local, national, and international story. In particular, I wish to acknowledge the 2010 Vancouver Winter Olympics Organization for giving me the honour to take part in the Torch Relay.

I wish to thank Alma Lee, founder of the Vancouver Writer's Festival, for carefully reading the third draft of the manuscript and for her encouragement and suggestions. I want to acknowledge Dr. Gloria McArter for her valuable insights regarding my story.

Ivana Cameron, exercise instructor in fitness, strength and energy offered her expert suggestions in drafting the OK exercises. Her input was invaluable in making these exercises effective and safe for seniors. Chris Shirley of the Pacific Institute of Reflexology kindly shared the hand and foot reflexology charts.

Thank you to graphic artist Carmen Lane for organizing the many photographs and to the editors at Friesen Press because these chapters became more appealing and readable after their input. Editing the work of others is not a simple task. Now I know what building a book really means.

Thanks to my nephew and his wife, Noris and Nora Burdeniuk, for the photography and their excellent photo editing skills. Thanks also to photographers Cindy Goodman for the exercise photos and Patrik Giardino http://www.giardinophoto.com for the California photographs that grace the beginning of each chapter.

I should like to thank the many persons who helped me by submitting to my endless questions or supporting this work. While I shall not attempt to record every debt here, I should particularly like to mention and thank Hugh McKinnon, Earl Fee, Ken Stone, Warren Hamill for their recommendations and encouragement.

A special thank you to Bishop Ken Nowakowski, who continually encourages me to extract and utilize my inner strength to keep my body, mind and spirit healthy and strong.

I thank sincerely Father Josephat, Pastor at Protection of the Blessed Virgin Mary Ukrainian Catholic Church Vancouver Parish; Mir

Huculak, lawyer, friend and Consul for Ukraine in Vancouver; and dear, cheerful and positive friend Theresa Herchak of Richmond for her letter of support.

Harold Morioka, coach, trainer of B.C. Fraser Valley Greyhounds Masters Track and Field Club for his patience and expertise in keeping track of my athletic competitions and especially my world records.

Dr. Tanja Taivassalo and her husband Dr. Russ Hepple, Professors in McGill's department of Kinesiology and Physical Education. Their research has focused on the pathophysiology of skeletal muscle mitochondrial disorders and the safety and efficacy of exercise training in their treatment. I am truly indebted for being included in the study.

Dr. Arthur Kramer and Dr. Laura Chaddock at the Beckman Institute at the University of Illinois for their patience and kindness while conducting their research on my brain.

Dr. Michael Myckatyn, a sincere thank you for being such a good friend and a great leader and organizer in the community. I feel privileged to have been included as an example of superior senior athleticism in the teaching sessions with your fellow doctors.

Barb Vida, thank you for enriching my life as a coach, trainer and a sincere friend. Her intense focus on determination, perseverance and commitment became powerful and influential in my sports career and has transferred into my personal healthy lifestyle. I still have the techniques and my experience, for which I am truly grateful.

Daniel Godfrey, Aqua Plus instructor at the West Vancouver Aquatic Centre has succeeded to make the high-intensity 60-minute workout fun for the class as he stresses endurance and strength building. My cardiovascular fitness has benefitted and increased in his energizing and motivating environment.

No project of any magnitude happens without sponsors and financial assistance. I wish to express my gratitude for the support and generosity of the Taras Shevchenko Foundation, who invest in the future of our Ukrainian community in Canada and maintain and strengthen our Canadian Ukrainian identity. I am so grateful that my book is a part of your generous support.

Senator Raynell Adreychuk noted that Canada would be a very different place today without the contribution of Ukrainian Canadians who worked hard to make this country so prosperous.

Gladys Andreas is a dear friend who has devoted her time and energy to promote and celebrate Ukrainian language, culture and customs to British Columbians.

Robert and Mary Lashin, their willingness and unequivocal eagerness to support my book brought it to fruition. Thank you.

Charles Taylor and his mechanics at North Vancouver Taylormotive merit a big thank you for their contribution toward the publications of this book and for keeping my 2000 Oldsmobile Intrigue in great working order. I really appreciate it.

Joseph and Annie Siermy, bass and alto singers in St Mary's choir, have generously extended support in bringing this book to completion. The gracious Lida Hoffman and Barbara Ballhorn generously give of their time and support to me and to St. Mary's Parish in the Cancer Society's Relay for Life. On behalf of my daughter Nadine I wish to congratulate our St Mary's team who continue to raise a lot of money towards cancer research.

Bruce Grierson, whose articles in *Reader's Digest, The New York Times Magazine,* and his book *What Makes Olga Run?* sent my life into a new direction. Right from the beginning, his unfailing guidance and support are gratefully acknowledged. My friend, thank you.

Stephanie Toporowski and Stephanie Dorosiewich, my dear, dear friends have given me so much of what is precious to me today.

Soloway Travel and Myrna Arychuk have been reuniting people with their relatives in Ukraine, Poland and Russia. Her *Solovei Magazine* will be promoting my book *Olga: The O.K. Way to a Healthy, Happy Life.*

Thanks to Millie Kozak, archivist, poet and devoted parishioner in the Holy Eucharist Ukrainian Catholic Cathedral in New Westminster. She researched and insisted that I include in this book only the best picture of the icon which I painted for the cathedral many years ago in 1968.

Anne Gutiw, Bernice Shawaga and Carol Issel, members of the younger generation for providing the document "Shawaga Family Reunion, 1901 – 1986". Thank you very much.

If I have forgotten anyone please know that in my heart I thank all of my family, friends and fellow athletes, young and old, who have cheered me on and have been so encouraging with their warm support. Above all I sincerely thank the good Lord for His guidance and in helping me to bring this book to fruition. It's tough to be so vulnerable in front of the whole world for the first time in my life, especially at the age of 95.

Athletic Achievements

GLOSSARY

For Overview of Track and Field Championships

Sprints
60m
100m
200m
400m
800m

Jumps
HJ - high jumps
LJ - long jumps
TJ - triple jump

Throws
SP -shot put
DT - discus throw

JT - javelin throw
HT - hammer throw
WT – weight throw

Other
WR - World record
CR - Canadian record
TP – throw pentathlon
WP – weight pentathlon
Sp - Sprints
M – meters
Sec - seconds

Overview of Track and Field Championships in 2004
85 years old

March 10 – 14
1st World Masters Athletics Indoor Championships,
Sindelfingen, Germany. *9 Gold*

Sp – 60m – 13.98 sec	HJ – 0.89m WR	SP – 5.81m WR
Sp – 200m – 52.68sec	LJ – 1.91m WR	DT – 13.91m WR
HT – 14.86m WR	WT – 7.56m WR	JT – 16.25m WR

May 8 – 9
Centennial Track and Field Meet,
Hillside Stadium, Kamloops B.C. *4 Gold*

Sp – 100m – 22.10sec	HJ – 0.85m WR
HT – 16.83m	DT – 13.70m

June 19 – 20
Pacific Invitational & B.C.A Masters Championships,
Langley, B.C. *8 Gold*

Sp – 100m – 22.16sec	HJ – 0.85m	SP – 5.66m
Sp – 200m – 49.84sec	LJ – 2.02m	DT – 14.36mWR
JT – 15.94m	HT – 16.16m	

June 26 - 27
Haywood Masters Classics U. of Oregon, Eugene, Oregon U.S.A. *9 Gold*

Sp - 100m - 21.84sec	HJ - 0.89m WR	SP - 5.77m
Sp - 200m - 50.44sec	LJ - 2.01m	DT - 14.20m
JT - 18.56m WR	HT - 17.49m	WT - 7.68m

July 17 - 18
Canadian Masters Athletic Association Track and Field Championships. Calgary, Alberta, Canada. *10 Gold*

Sp – 100m – 21.83 sec	HJ – 0.85m	JT – 16.94m
Sp – 200m – 52.07 sec	LJ – 2.13m	HT – 17m
SP – 85.5m	DT – 14.55m	WT – 7.72m WR
Throws Pentathlon – 4211 points		

Aug 5 - 8
37th Annual USATF National Masters Championships, Decatur Illinois, U.S.A. *7 Gold*

Sp - 100m - 22.70sec	DT - 14.25m WR	HT - 16.67m
Sp - 200m - 55.81sec	LJ - 2.04m	JT - 15.70m
SP - 5.61m		

Olga Kotelko

Aug 27 - 29
NCCWMA T & F
Dorado, Puerto Rico. *11 Gold*

Sp - 100m - 22.19sec	HJ - 0.94m WR	SP - 5.94m WR
SP - 200m - 50.89sec	LJ - 2.11m	DT – 14.64m
HT - 16.57m	JT - 15.62m	Women 80 + Relay - 4x100m - 1:53:85sec WR
Sp - 400m - 2:28:07sec	Throws Pentathlon - 4391 points	

Sept. 1 - 4
B.C. Seniors Games,
Penticton, Canada. *8 Gold*

Sp – 100m – 21.18 sec	HJ – 0.85m	HT – 18.62m WR
Sp - 200m – 48.36 sec WR	SP – 5.68m	DT – 13.26m
	LJ – 2.01m	WT – 7.0m
Throws Pentathlon – 4280 points		

Oct 1 - 3
Nevada 2004 Senior Olympics, Univ. of Nevada,
Las Vegas, Nevada, U.S.A. *7 Gold*

Sp – 100m – 22.01 sec	HJ – 0.88m	SP – 6.03m WR
Sp – 200m – 52.01 sec	LJ – 1.84m	HT – 16.85m
Throws Pentathlon – 4442 points WR		

Oct 4 – 6

Hunts man World Seniors Games,

St. George, Utah, U.S.A. *6 Gold*

Sp – 100m – 21.95sec	HJ – 0.85m	SP – 6.03m
Sp – 200m – 52.30sec	LJ – 2.01m	DT – 14.61m

Total = 79 Gold

Overview of Track & Field Championships in 2009
90 years old

May 23 – 24

B.C. Masters Track and Field Championships,

Nanaimo, B.C. *10 Gold*

Sp – 100m – 22.02 sec	HJ – 0.75m WR	SP – 4.96m
WT – 6.54m WR	LJ – 1.58m WR	DT – 14.58m WR
TJ – 3.93m WR	JT – 13.31m WR	HT – 13.31m WR
Sp – 200m – 1:04:16 sec		

July 17 - 19
CMAA T & F Championships,
Kamloops, B.C. Canada. *5 Gold*

Sp - 100m - 27.87sec	HJ - 0.75m	TJ - 4.14m
LJ - 1.70m	Throws Pentathlon - 5878 points	

July 26 - Aug 08
WMA 2009 Championships,
Lahti, Finland. *11 Gold*

Sp - 100m - 25.05sec	HJ - 0.82m WR	DT - 14.80m
Sp - 200m - 56.46sec WR	LJ - 1.77m WR	SP - 4.86m
JT - 13.54m WR	HT - 12.92m	WT - 6.49m
Throws Pentathlon - 5905 points		TJ - 4.02m WR

Sept. 16 - 19
B.C. Seniors Games,
Richmond, B.C. Canada. *7 Gold*

Sp - 100m - 24.60sec	HJ - 0.80m	SP - 4.51m
Sp - 400m - 2:50:28sec WR	LJ - 1.46m	TJ - 4.25m WR
Throws Pentathlon - 5515 points		

Oct 10 - 18

World Masters Games,

Olympic Park, Sydney Australia *9 Gold*

DT – 13.42m	LJ – 1.72m	SP – 5.64m WR
TJ – 4.25m WR	JT – 12.51m	HT – 17.11m WR
WT – 8.04m WR	Throws Pentathlon – 6306 points WR	
Sp – 100m – 23.95sec WR		

Total = 42 Gold

"According to the statistics of the B.C. Masters Outdoor Track and Field Records by B.C. Master Record Director Harold Morioka, new records set in 2009 (as of December 01, 2009) show that Olga Kotelko (W90) has broken WR's 30, CR's 47 and BC records 47 times. Olga has set-broke "new" 10 WR's , 12 CR's and 12 B.C. records. Amazing! What an achievement for a 90 year-old female athlete.

"This was the first time ever that a 90 year-old female athlete jumped 3 jumps – high jump (0.82m), long jump (1.77m) and triple jump (4.25m) – quite an amazing standard. Every jump obviously is a World Record".

(For an athlete to get one World Record in a lifetime is an accomplishment.)

Hammer Throw is my favorite event. I want to show you what fun I have throwing the hammer.

Hammer Throw – when 4 years older I threw
2.49m farther (W85–89) 2007 – 88 years old

XVI WMA Riccioni, Italy – Hammer Throw
14.22m (W90–94) 2009 – 90 years old

WMA Games, Sydney, Australia – Hammer
Throw – 17.11m (W90–94) 2011 – 92 years old

WMA T&F Championships, Sacramento,
California – Hammer Throw 16.71m

Not too shabby! As of today, December 2, 2013, medal total is 717 gold, 26 silver, 8 bronze.

Interviews

I was dazed and overwhelmed by all the attention and affection coming my way since *The New York Times Magazine* published the article "The Incredible Flying Nonagenarian" in November 28, 2010 written by Bruce Grierson. This media experience was not exactly easy. However I persisted and carried on forward. It was the most different period in my life. I might have missed acknowledging some of my appointments and I apologize. To date I am still involved periodically with the media.

Television

CBC – National News Nov. 29, 2010 with Peter Mansbridge.

CBC "As it Happens" show.

BBC – World News.

America BC Global News 2010.

Ellen DeGeneres Talk Show, Dec. 2, 2010 (phone interview).

Ukrainian National TV.

Ukrainian TV (local private).

Globo LTDA Brazil, Apr.2011 promoting 2014 World Cup Soccer and 2016 Brazilian Olympic Games.

Shaw TV.

Documentary profile "My Vancouver" on Telus.

Optik TV Globo Brazil October 2013 "Fantastico".

Canada AM – Toronto January 16, 2014.

NBC Today Show – January 17, 2014.

Radio

CBC – Radio, Toronto, Nov. 29, 6:00 p.m.

WMFE – Orlando Florida, "The Growing Bolder" show.

NPR – National Public Radio, Boston Dec. 3, 8a.m.

CBC – "Afternoon Edition" Regina, Saskatchewan, Friday Dec.3, 3p.m.

CBC – Toronto Documentary, Sept. 2011.

CBC – "Q" with Jian Ghomeshi January 2014.

Magazines

The New York Times Magazine, "The Incredible Flying Nonagenarian". Bruce Grierson, Nov. 28, 2010 Page 72.

Hello! Canada Magazine, "World in Pictures" Nov. 9, 2009.

McGill University, Study and Research, "The Gazette Montreal"
Apr. 23, 2010.

Zoomer Magazine, "She's ONE at 91" Apr.10, 2010, Page 130.

Reader's Digest, "Olga the Athlete", Bruce Grierson, May 2010, Page 25.

Great Britain *Stella* Magazine/ *The Sunday Telegraph*, London, Page 34 "Nonagenarian Nonpariel" Jan. 2, 2011. [hmmm, not bad for 91]

Headway "McGill Research, Discovery and Innovations. "The Aging Issue" Summer 2011 Page 8.

Vancouver Magazine, "125 Reasons to Love This City" June 20, 2011, Page 64.

McGill News - Alumni Magazine - fall/winter 2012 Page 40, (2nd row, bottom middle picture, with Mike Babcock.)

Numerous Health and Wellness Magazines.

Health Action "Breaking Records at 93: Olga Kotelko" Summer 2012.

Parade Magazine – Sunday December 29, 2014.

Reader's Digest – January 2014.

Newspapers

The Vancouver Sun, The Province, North Shore News, B.C. Catholic, North Shore Outlook, Saskatoon Star Phoenix and local newspapers wherever I competed.

Major German Daily - *Suddeutache Zeitung* Nr.285/Donners, 9 Dezember/Seite 9 "The Best Track and Field Athlete in the World - in her age group".

LeMonde - Sport & Forme - French National Newspaper. "la grand mere aus 600 medailles d'or", Jan. 7 2012, "Mamie Olympique ".

Finish Newspaper Daily.

Metro Birmingham England (shot put).

Argentina Newspaper Daily.

Toronto Sunday Media "Spectacular Seniors".

Australia Newspaper Daily.

Leader Post "Senior Track Stars Beating the Clock" June 11, 2012.

Zero Hora - Local newspaper Porto Alegre, Brazil October 2013.

Others

Olympic Torch Relay, Vancouver 2010 Winter Olympics Study and Research, McGill University, Department of Kinesiology, Physical Education, 2010, 2012.

Illinois Beckman Institute, Chicago, 2012.

Autumn Gold Film – *Herbstgold* = German Documentary Film 2013.

Recognition by Dawn Black, MP – New Westminster – Coquitlam 2009.

Master Female, Track and Field Athlete of the Year award Documentary producer Brandy Yanchyk due July 2014.

IPA Metodista University Porto Alegre, Brazil – Journalism October 2013.

West Vancouver Sorority Club - October 18, 2013.

Vancouver Toastmasters Club – November 7, 2013.

The Huffington Post – telephone interview.

Senior Living Magazine September 24, 2013.

Note: I am unable to list absolutely everything; I missed a few.

Bibliography

The Family Guide to Reflexology, By Ann Gillanders Little, Brown and Company. Boston, New York, Toronto, London.

Fitness For Seniors, Amazing Body Breakthroughs for Super Health. By Frank St. Carwood and Associates. Inc. 103 Clover Green Peachtree City GA.

Pilates for Fragile Backs, By Andra Fischgrund Stanton, With Ruth Hiatt-Coblentz. New Harbinger Publication Inc. www.newharbinger.com.

Getting in Shape, The Basic Program 5 by Bob Anderson Shelter Publications. Inc.

Awakening the Spine, The Stress-free new yoga that works with the body to restore health, vitality and energy. By Vanda Scaravelli. Harper, San Francisco.

Water Fitness, Lesson Plans and Choreography Christine Alexander. Human Kinetics ©2011 by Christine Alexander.

The Complete Aquatic Fitness Guide Phys Ex, Believe in your Abilities. Produced and written by Sandra Starrett, B.P.E ©2008 Physical Expressions.

The Oil Protein Diet Cookbook Dr. Johanna Budwig. Apple Publishing Co. Ltd.

Healthy Eating For Seniors Senior BC. British Columbia publication. Foreward: P.R.W Kendall MBBS, MSc, FRCPC Provincial Health Officer.

Growing Younger - Breakthrough age-defying secrets for women, By Bridget Doherty, Julia Van Tine and the Editors of Prevention Health Book for Women 2002 Rodale Inc U.S.A.

The Core Program - Fifteen Minutes a Day that can change your life By Peggy W. Brill, PT, With Gerald S. Couzens Bantam Books.

The Joy of Cooking. Irma S. Rombauer and Marion Rombauer Becker The Bobbs-Merrill Co. Inc. Indianapolis, Indiana U.S.A.

Meaning and Medicine Dr. Larry Dossey.

Generations of Faith Programme of the Ukrainian Churches Catholic and Orthodox, "Christian Symbolism of Paschal Foods in the Ukrainian Tradition".

Traditional Ukrainian Cookery Savella Stechishin Trident Press, Ltd. Winnipeg, MB.

Ukrainian Traditional and Modern Cuisine Published by Eparchial Executive. Ukrainian Catholic Women's League of Canada Eparchy of New Westminster, BC, Canada Yavoslava Tatarniuk, Olga Kotelko.

From the author

As a teacher, nothing gave me greater pleasure than to observe the look of comprehension that came over my students' faces when I saw that they had learned an important lesson, something of value that might benefit them for the rest of their lives. What I have learned and experienced over my long life may help you, too, achieve the same physical, mental, and spiritual benefits I enjoy. This is not a memoir as I didn't want to stay trapped in never-ending nostalgia. I want people who read my story to believe that it is possible to embark on the road to health—one firm step at a time—by starting to move in the direction of well-being.

CPSIA information can be obtained at www.ICGtesting.com
Printed in the USA
LVOW11*2335280816

502228LV00002B/17/P